PLAGUE, QUARANTINES AND GEOPOLITICS IN THE OTTOMAN EMPIRE

PLAGUE, QUARANTINES AND GEOPOLITICS IN THE OTTOMAN EMPIRE

✦ ✦ ✦

BİRSEN BULMUŞ

EDINBURGH
University Press

For my mother, Beyaz Bulmuş and my late father, Ahmet Bulmuş

Edinburgh University Press Ltd
22 George Square, Edinburgh EH8 9LF
www.euppublishing.com

Typeset in JaghbUni Regular by
Servis Filmsetting Ltd, Stockport, Cheshire, and
printed and bound in Great Britain by
CPI Group (UK) Ltd, Croydon CR0 4YY

A CIP record for this book is available from the British Library

ISBN 978 0 7486 4659 3 (hardback)
ISBN 978 0 7486 4660 9 (webready PDF)
ISBN 978 0 7486 5547 2 (epub)
ISBN 978 0 7486 5546 5 (Amazon ebook)

CONTENTS

Acknowledgements vi

Map showing the Ottoman Empire, 1914 viii

1. PRELIMINARY REMARKS 1
2. CONCEPTUALISING PLAGUE IN OTTOMAN ISLAMIC THOUGHT 15
3. PLAGUE AND OTTOMAN MEDICAL THOUGHT 39
4. MAGIC AND PLAGUE IN THE OTTOMAN EMPIRE 68
5. HAMDAN BIN EL-MERHUM OSMAN AND THE OTTOMAN QUARANTINE REFORM 97
6. PLAGUE AND QUARANTINES IN THE COLONIAL ERA 130
7. PLAGUE, SANITARY ADMINISTRATION AND THE END OF EMPIRE 152
8. TOWARDS A NEW UNDERSTANDING OF PLAGUE AND QUARANTINES IN THE OTTOMAN EMPIRE 177

Bibliography 181

Index 191

ACKNOWLEDGEMENTS

This book is the product of many years of labour, and evolved out of my PhD thesis, 'Plague in the Ottoman Empire, 1300–1838', which I completed at the Department of History, Georgetown University in May 2008. I would have not completed my work without the encouragement of my mentor, Dr Kathy Olesko, and that of the other members of my PhD dissertation committee, Dr John O. Voll and Dr Carol Benedict. I have also been guided by a wide range of scholars in Ottoman, Middle Eastern and European history, Turkish studies and historical sociology. These include: Dr Sandra Horvath-Peterson, Georgetown University; Dr Özkul Çobanoğlu, Hacettepe University; Dr Kelvin A. Santiago-Valles, Binghamton University; Dr Halil İnalcık, world-renowned scholar and my great MA mentor at Bilkent University; and Dr Ali Doğramacı, Rector of Bilkent University. I also feel an enormous debt of gratitude to Dr Farhan Ahmad Nizami, director at Centre for Islamic Studies and Dr Eugene L. Rogan, Faculty of Oriental Studies, University of Oxford, for their assistance following my visit to Oxford in the summer of 1996.

I have also been the beneficiary of support from a number of research institutions, whose help was absolutely critical to the successful completion of my book. These include the Ankara University Faculty of Divinity Library, Atatürk Library, Devlet Library, Hacı Selim Ağa Rare Manuscript Library, Millet Rare Manuscript Library, National Library, Religious Affairs Library, Süleymaniye Library, T. C. Prime Ministry State Archives, Turkish Religious Foundation Centre for Islamic Studies (İSAM) and Turkish Historical Society Library, all in Ankara and Istanbul, Turkey. I also benefited greatly from collections at the Georgetown University Library, Library of Congress, National Library of Medicine, University of Wisconsin-Madison Libraries and New York Public

Library. I would like to thank several librarians and related officials, particularly Servet Arıtürk, İstanbul Metropolitan Municipality; Salih Gülen, Editor and Chief of *Hazine Yayınları*; Ebubekir Kaya, İstanbul University Central Library; Erdem Selçuk, Beyazıt State Library; Perihan Sezen, İstanbul University Medical School Hulusi Behçet Library; and Mustafa Birol Ülker, Director of the Turkish Religious Foundation Centre for Islamic Studies. I am also very grateful to Crystal Smith and Karen Pitts from the National Library of Medicine, Washington, DC.

I have also benefited recently from continuous feedback from my friends, especially my fellow colleagues in the Department of History at Appalachian State University, particularly Dr Lucinda McCray, who shares a common interest in the history of medicine, Dr James Goff, Dr Tim Silver and Dr Michael Wade. I also have gained much encouragement in recent months from Mehmet Ali Akat of Paterson, New Jersey and Orçun Temizkan of Charlotte, North Carolina. Mohamed Ben Yahia of Fairfax, Virginia has also been a great friend and has provided generous time in reading relevant Arabic texts related to my project.

In addition, I would especially like to thank Dr York Norman of Buffalo State College for his generous support during all stages of this project, including his patient editing of my work and his translations of relevant materials from Bosnian and German to English.

I am also very grateful to Dr Nancy Gallagher of the University of California-Santa Barbara and Dr Colin Imber of the University of Manchester for their reviews of my work.

Nicola Ramsey, Senior Commissioning Editor, and her colleagues at Edinburgh University Press were ultimately also key to the successful completion of the book.

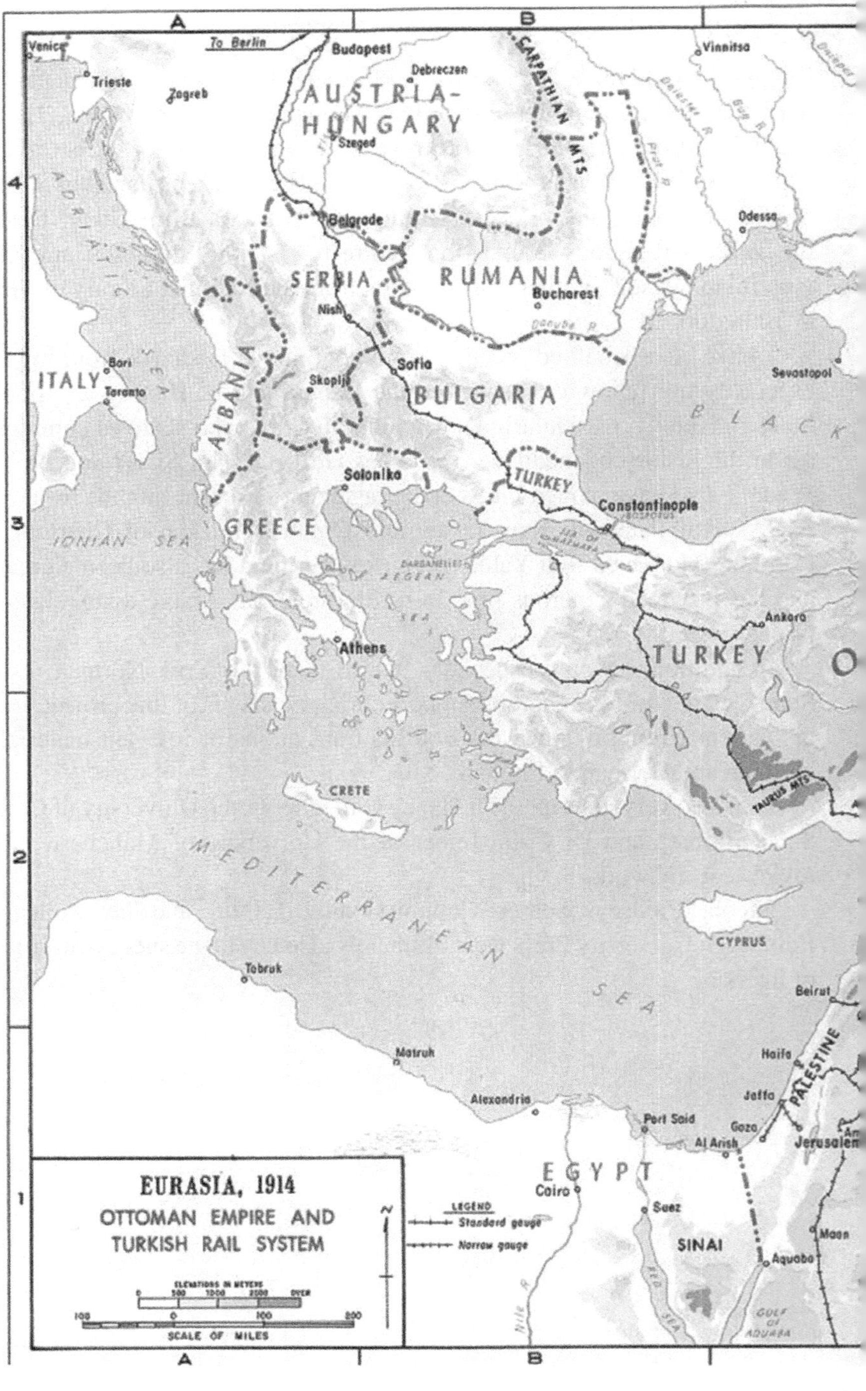

Map showing the Ottoman Empire, 1914 (United States Military Academy)

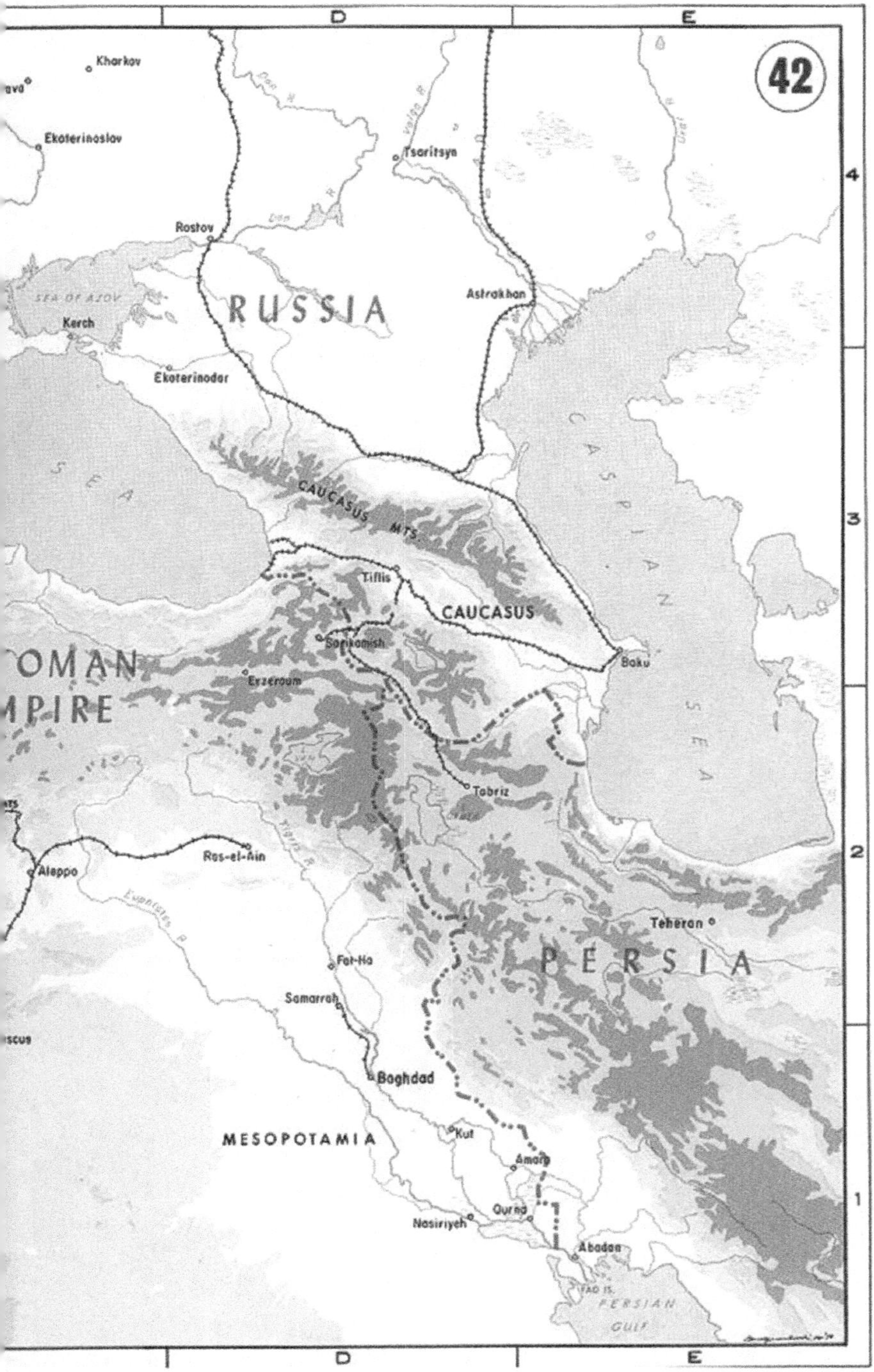
42
D
E
4
3
2
1
Kharkov
Ekaterinoslav
Tsaritsyn
Volga R.
Don R.
Rostov
SEA OF AZOV
Kerch
RUSSIA
Astrakhan
Ekaterinodar
CAUCASUS MTS.
CASPIAN SEA
Tiflis
CAUCASUS
Sarikamish
Baku
OMAN
MPIRE
Erzeroum
Tabriz
Ras-el-Ain
Aleppo
Tigris R.
Euphrates R.
Teheran
PERSIA
Fat-Ha
Samarrah
Baghdad
MESOPOTAMIA
Kut
Amara
Qurna
Nasiriyeh
Abadan
FAO IS.
PERSIAN GULF

CHAPTER

1

PRELIMINARY REMARKS

One day in the summer of 2004 I wandered down to the shores of Istanbul's Golden Horn and saw a peculiar sight: a grand, yellow, nineteenth-century building sitting directly on top of one of the district's most famous mosques. Right next to it was an equally elegant red-brown office, directly on the shores of the bay. International travellers to the city who come by boat have to go to these buildings even today in order to undergo medical inspection to see if they have contracted any epidemic disease. Certainly, most travellers to Istanbul before the mid-twentieth century would almost certainly have been familiar with the compound, as ships were the mode of overseas travel.

After learning from the guards that the buildings were constructed in the mid-nineteenth century, I, as a student of the history of medicine in the Middle East, wondered why the Ottomans had waited so long. Travellers began to complain of plague spreading from the district's docks to the surrounding city shortly after Sultan Mehmed II's conquest of the city in 1453, and yet it took about 400 years for a quarantine to be built. I wondered, then, to what extent geopolitical and cultural influences explained this development.

I remembered that the Ottomans essentially remained a premodern state until Napoleon's conquest of Egypt in 1798 forced the Sultanate to embark on modernising reform in order to save the empire from disintegration. Istanbul and the realm's other major port cities had relatively few Muslim merchants and a comparatively weak navy, and relied on non-Muslims and foreigners to develop their overseas trade. The result was a lack of both a politically conscious Muslim middle class and a lively press culture that expressed interest in modernising reform and economic development.

I had the impression from the Ottoman primary sources that I looked at over the next few months that the Istanbul quarantine facility was one of many innovations partially inspired by the Europeans. Anton Lago, an Austrian doctor who worked for the Ottoman Sultan Muhmud II, wrote a famous work in 1836 that argued that the Ottomans should construct the quarantine facilities. Like most European advocates of quarantine until that time, Lago maintained that the plague was an ether-like substance that spread to humans either by person-to-person contact or by exposure to plague-infested materials such as wool and cotton. I also realised that Ottoman writers centuries before Lago's time were aware of the European experience with epidemic disease. İlyas bin Abram Al-Yahudi (d. 1513), a Jewish refugee who fled from the Reconquista to offer services to the Ottoman court, wrote a medical treatise on his experience with the plague in Spain. İdris-i Bitlisi (d. 1520) similarly wrote about how the Europeans used mercury to cure the plague and urged his Ottoman audience to do the same.[1]

Europeans had also written extensively about plague in the Ottoman Empire. A number of key English authors blamed the great plague of London in 1665 and the 1720 Marseille outbreak on unregulated imports of plague-infested cotton and wool. These accusations helped to justify the construction of quarantines by the late sixteenth century that not only guarded borders against disease, but also gave their sovereigns greater control over foreign trade and any monopolies associated with it. The quarantine had the potential to help to promote domestic production in the name of public health and, thus, could be of great institutional importance in promoting mercantilism. Quarantine reform was also often used to categorise certain groups that were more likely to spread the plague. These reforms empowered state officials to medically police the poor and immigrant populations in thriving port cities like London from the sixteenth to the early twentieth centuries.[2]

Until 1838, British critics of these measures pointed to the Ottoman Empire as a positive example, since there was no quarantine there. In their opinion, the quarantine and sanitary police were cruel and unnecessary measures that hindered trade and humiliated many. It was no coincidence that liberal British writers would condemn the Ottomans after 1838 for repeating their own 'mistake'.[3]

I still wondered, however, whether there was more to this story of the Ottoman quarantine than simply Mahmud II's acceptance of Lago's European-style quarantine in 1838. I had also read the treatise of Hamdan Bin El-Merhum Osman Hoca (1773–1840), a contemporary of Lago who also wrote a key text in 1836 advocating quarantine reform to the sultan. Hamdan, an Algerian notable who fled to the Ottoman Empire in the wake of the French occupation, was mainly concerned with convincing Muslim elites within the empire about the necessity of the reform.[4]

One key argument for Hamdan was that the new institution was fully justified according to Islam. He often referred to earlier Ottoman plague treatise writers. These included famous sixteenth-century figures. Bitlisi vigorously defended his avoidance of plague in Damascus after performing his ritual pilgrimage to Mecca in 1512 from his critics. Ebussuud Efendi (1491–1574), the single most influential Ottoman Islamic jurist of the sixteenth century, also supported flight from plague as a justifiable precaution. Bitlisi and Ebussuud – and Hamdan – could also cite pre-Ottoman Islamic thinkers to support their opinions. They would at times mention Lisaneddin Al-Khattib (d. 1375), an Islamic scholar who advocated medical precautions after witnessing the 1348 outbreak of the Black Death, and the famous Sufi mystic, Abu Hamid Ghazali (1058–1111), who wrote of the need for human compassion for plague victims. They would reference Caliph Umar (634–44), who also fled the plague, as well as selected sayings of Muhammad, to justify their positions. In addition, Hamdan cited earlier Ottoman medical treatises on plague that justified medical treatment. Such earlier works not only dealt with flight – the most controversial of topics during the sixteenth century – but also with prescriptions and fumigation. These treatments often paralleled those of premodern European medical writers on plague.[5]

Hamdan was different from many of these earlier writers in at least one key respect: he did not ever view plague in mystical terms and shunned the use of magic or ritual prayer to ward off the disease. Writers like Bitlisi, Ebussuud Efendi and Kemaleddin Taşköprüzade (d. 1621) included such elements within their treatises as one of many ways to fight the disease. Ahmed Efendi Müneccimbaşı bin Halil er-Rumi (d. 1748) had gone so far as to write an entire work on plague and the elemental magic of talismans in 1667–8.[6] Hamdan, like most modern European plague reformers, abandoned magic in favour of empirically proven scientific principles.

One European innovation that Hamdan did not introduce was the use of quarantine as a social disciplinary tool to police the poor or other subject groups. Hamdan, like Turhan Pasha (d. 1914), a later Ottoman medical reformer, may have opposed the measure out of religious conviction, as such policing treated segments of the population as virtual subhumans. It is also quite likely that he recognised that medical policing might lead to authoritarian tendencies in government: a problem for the Europeans who first developed the sanitary police.[7] In fact, no major Ottoman quarantine official embraced discriminatory measures until 1894 – including the famous former chiefs Ahmed Midhat (1844–1912) and Besim Ömer (1862–1940).

Hamdan and his audience were concerned about increasing foreign penetration. While many Muslims were afraid that the Ottoman Empire might share Algeria's fate as a colony, others pointed to the increasing influence of

British and French loans and commercial influence, while yet others pointed to European support of Muhammad Ali of Egypt (1769–1849) as a rival to their own sultan. Hamdan implied that quarantine would help to defend Ottoman sovereignty in resisting these tendencies. Quarantine could potentially assist the native textile producers by controlling British and other European imports as 'suspected goods', affording the Ottoman authorities the possibility of taxing or even banning these goods.[8]

Unsurprisingly, the Europeans – particularly the British – protested that the establishment of the Ottoman quarantine in 1838 was clearly contrary to the Ottomans commitment to free trade. Lord Ponsonby (1770–1855), the British ambassador to the Sublime Porte, having imposed the Balta Liman unequal trade agreement on the Ottomans that year, succeeded in forming the Constantinople Superior Health Council, an international body, to supervise the quarantine. The British would also prompt other major European powers to gather a series of international sanitary conferences to which the Ottoman quarantine would also be subject. As these developments indicate, the Ottoman and foreign governments would struggle during the ensuing eighty years over who would ultimately control the quarantine, its policies and revenues.

The French and British reacted to the 1838 Ottoman quarantine by embracing a new understanding of plague as infectious in places where filthy and unhygienic conditions propagated the disease. This understanding, pioneered by French doctors Antoine Clot (1793–1868) and Louis Aubert-Roche (1810–74) in Egypt in 1841, was in contrast to the previous view of plague as being spread from person to person or through infected goods. They advocated increased medical policing of at-risk populations, such as Egypt, India, China and the Ottoman Empire – all non-European countries. Advocates of this new school of thought argued that the Ottoman quarantine was not enough to get rid of the disease. They supposed that only the Europeans themselves had the means and technological know-how to improve sanitation, building codes, sewage and water supply systems in order to transform the infested areas into hygienic living space. These views helped to justify colonial control of public health in Egypt, often humiliating the native population as coming from an inferior, diseased culture.[9] The British institutionalised these practices in Egypt's major cities and in medical inspection stations set up along the Suez Canal after they declared Egypt a protectorate in 1882.

The British and French held a number of international sanitary conferences in 1892, 1894, 1897 and 1903 to institutionalise medical inspection procedures with regard to the annual Muslim pilgrimage to Mecca. The Europeans claimed the pilgrimage routes – often with crowds of over 100,000 pilgrims per year – were unsanitary and spread plague and cholera. Many of the pilgrims were from colonised countries, and the ruling European powers believed that the colonisers and the colonised were both at risk. The Europeans sought strict regulations on the pilgrim traffic. Every pilgrim would not only have to pre-pay his or her ticket, but would also have to undergo a series of medical inspections at the Suez Canal and along the Red Sea, and also before and after departure to the Hijaz, the Ottoman province of western Arabia.[10] Alexandre Yersin's discovery of the bubonic plague bacilli as the biological cause of plague in 1894 only slightly changed these regulations to include inspection and fumigation for rats and rat-infested materials. The medical officials at the time believed unhygienic conditions and poor sanitation were responsible for spreading plague from rats and fleas to human populations.

The conferences did not resolve the underlying political tensions between the Ottomans and the European powers. The British, in control of the Suez Canal, the sea lanes and major shipping companies, gained greater leverage over distant Ottoman territory, leading Muslims to question whether the Empire retained its sovereignty as the premier Sunni Muslim state. The Europeans also had political considerations in mind. Knowing that Sultan Abdulhamid II (r. 1876–1909) promoted a message of pan-Islamist unity in the face of European colonialism, they feared that colonial subjects who visited might be incited to rebel at home.

Kasim İzzeddin (1859–1926), the leader of the Ottoman sanitation effort after 1894, made the fateful decision to adopt medical inspection methods. In contrast to Hamdan and his successors, İzzeddin would not only maintain maritime quarantines in the major ports of the Ottoman Empire, he would also oversee new urban plans, construct new water supplies, sewage systems, hospitals, urban shelters and – very importantly – police the poor and the pilgrims.

İzzeddin's reforms targeted two critical frontier districts: the Hijaz, home to Mecca and Medina; and southern Iraq, where the Ottomans oversaw an annual pilgrimage of Shia Muslims from Persia and Russia. These efforts embittered the relationship of the Ottoman central authority with local populations. Both the Bedouins of the Hijaz and the Shia of southern Iraq felt that they were being systematically discriminated against, and may well have questioned the value of their continued loyalty to the Ottoman state. İzzeddin, a Lebanese Sunni Muslim who also feared foreign encroachment of the Arab lands of the Ottoman Empire, thought that centralisation through sanitation reform would help to consolidate Ottoman rule once railway lines had connected Mecca, Baghdad and Basra to the main Ottoman grid.[11] Oddly enough, these efforts won considerable international support, particularly from the British. İzzeddin and the Ottomans would be dependent on British coal, machinery and transportation and this increased British leverage in these frontier areas; at least until the railway was established, when these materials could be sent over land and not by sea through British-dominated waters.

After November 1914, when the Ottoman and British empires found themselves at war, the British cut off this technical and logistical support, and İzzeddin's efforts were doomed to failure. The local Bedouin population rebelled in the Hijaz, and the Shia of southern Iraq put up no major resistance against the British when they invaded in 1916.

After the First World War and the brief British occupation of Istanbul and the Straits, Atatürk and the new Turkish Republic asserted its control over the quarantine facilities in Turkey. The new regime abolished all foreign oversight, but kept its administrative headquarters in the Golden Horn complex I first saw.[12]

This book will elaborate on the long and intricate geopolitical history of plague, national sovereignty and quarantine in the Ottoman Empire from 1300 until the end of the First World War by delving into the writings of the main actors in this drama. These treatise writers included not only Hamdan and his contemporaries, but also other Ottoman thinkers and statesmen throughout this time period. I will additionally consider works by British, French and other pertinent Western travellers, doctors, diplomats and scholars that influenced or were analogous to Ottoman conceptions of plague and the quarantine and sanitary reform movement.

Indeed, historians have highlighted plague's role in the rise and fall of empires and states in the Middle East and eastern Mediterranean. As Lawrence Conrad has shown, the first outbreak of plague occurred in 541–2 during the time of the Byzantine emperor Justinian, and had a devastating impact on the sedentary population of the fertile crescent, key to maintaining Constantinople's rule in the area. Plague deaths in major cities like Antioch and their grain-producing hinterland weakened the Byzantines' economic and military ability to retain the province. The Byzantines soon came to rely upon the trading and military skills of the Bedouin, who moved into the area from the nearby Arabian Peninsula. The Bedouin, like the Ottoman Turks nearly seven centuries later, would use their predatory skills to found an empire of their own. The early Islamic empire, founded by Muhammad and his companions, would dominate the region until the end of the Umayyad dynasty in 750. Oddly enough, a second great outbreak of plague may well have hastened the end of the dynasty, since the newly entrenched Arab elites in Damascus had themselves become sedentarised and therefore more vulnerable to an epidemic.[13]

The importance of plague to the rise of the Islam, as Conrad illustrates, can even be seen in the Quran itself. In the 105th chapter, *Al-Fil* (The Elephant), the Quran talks about the fate of an Abyssinian army that sought to subject Mecca and take over the Kaba on the eve of Muhammad's birth:[14]

> Hast thou not seen the people of the elephant, how dealt with them the Lord? Did not He make their plot to end in ruin abhorred? When He sent against them birds, horde on horde, and stones of baked clay upon them poured, and made them as leaves of corn devoured.

Conrad postulates that these lines are, in fact, a metaphorical reference to an outbreak of plague that was visited upon the Abyssinians by divine intervention, an immediate sign of God's presence in history. The common traditional Muslim attribution of plague to the work of angel-like genies (*jinn*), and the view that those who died from plague were martyrs to God also coincides with this belief.

Yet Conrad also demonstrates that Muhammad and his companions sometimes advocated taking physical precautions to avoid the disease. Muhammad commanded at one point that 'if it (plague) is in a land, do not enter it'. He also alluded to flight as an option to avoid contagious disease when he instructed the faithful to 'flee from the leper, as you would flee from a lion'. Admittedly, Muhammad made other injunctions to the contrary, positing that there was no contagion, that one should not leave a plague-infested area, and that God was the ultimate cause of disease. Still, all of these statements need to be put in their proper context. Conrad points out, for example, that Muhammad's assertion of 'no contagion' was likely part of a broad condemnation of nature worshipers, who saw contagious disease as divine.[15] Conrad shows that popular beliefs in contagion continued to persist, stating: 'the Umayyad poet Jarir sang of a "spreading contagion quickly communicated [to others]", while his rival Farazdag spoke of how "contact with her infects the healthy".'[16]

This ambivalent attitude towards contagious disease was most famously displayed after the outbreak of plague in Amwas, a town near Damascus, where, in 638, Abu Ubaydah, one of Caliph Umar's commanding generals, was ordered to leave the vicinity to go to the more distant town of Serag after plague was discovered in the area. Ubaydah argued against fleeing, saying it was God's will for him to stay. Umar then told him through a parable that God had ordained that he should take precautions:

> Yes, we are fleeing from the will of God, to the will of God . . . Suppose you have camels which come into a valley with two slopes, one lush with pasturage and the other barren; if you graze them on the lush slopes, would that not be by the will of God, and if you graze them on the barren slope, would that not also be by the will of God?[17]

Authors from this time onwards would cite this exchange as demonstrating the righteousness of their cause. Those who argued for precaution referred to Umar's parable, his leadership as caliph and the fact that Abu Ubaydah ultimately obeyed his command. Others countered that Abu Ubaydah's initial protest was valid, and that he in fact regretted obeying Umar.

My work is aimed in large part at explaining this tension throughout Ottoman history, following Conrad's call for greater elaboration on the subject: 'To assert that "Islam" denies contagion is therefore to miss the essence of what was in fact a complex and difficult debate that has continued through most of Islamic history, involving contributions by individuals too numerous to consider here.'[18]

Conrad's work is also influential for establishing that early Muslim physicians differentiated plague from other contagious diseases. According to Imam Nawawi (1234–78): 'Every plague (*taun*) is a pestilence (*waba*), but not every pestilence is a plague.'[19] To Conrad, early Islamic physicians saw *taun* as a physical reference to buboes, a clear proof that the disease was indeed bubonic plague, whose biological agent was discovered by Alexander Yersin and Kitasato Shibasaburo in Hong Kong in 1894.

Yersina pestis was a seemingly harmless non-motile cell that, in the right conditions, quickly and uncontrollably reproduced in the warm, moist blood of its victims. The bacilli was largely confined to populations of black rats (*rattus rattus*), which Conrad argues were prevalent in the premodern Middle East both in urban areas and their agricultural hinterlands. Moreover, fleas, particularly the variety *Xenopsylla cheopis*, which was particularly fond of black rat blood, had a tendency to pass on *Yersina pestis* to other rats. Although *Yersina pestis* almost always peacefully co-existed with its rat and flea hosts, rare outbreaks of the disease could occur. When they did, *x. cheopis* fleas became particularly virulent, as the *Yersina pestis* gathered and multiplied in its black rat blood-filled stomach. This would 'block' the flea from swallowing more food, making it bite its victims much more frequently, dramatically increasing the chance it could pass on the disease. While for most of the time the affected rat population was isolated from humans, disaster would strike when people came into close proximity with infected fleas, as flea bites were the most common means of contracting the plague. *Yersina pestis* would then grow uncontrollably in the bloodstream, where its gel-like shell prevented it from being eaten by 'the human body's normal defences', the bacilli-eating phagocytes.[20]

If the body's lymphatic system carried the *Yersina pestis* cells to exterior lymph nodes, 'the hordes of bacilli collected in these nodes and created a case of bubonic plague with characteristic swellings or "buboes" in the groin and armpits and behind the ear', reflective of an unrestricted growth of cells that usually killed the victim within six to eight days.[21] If the bulk of the *Yersina pestis* were instead transmitted to interior lymphatic nodes, as was usual in 5–15 per cent of cases, the victim would die from septicemic plague without swellings, as the cells would quickly would block the circulatory system, fatally damaging the heart and other vital organs. Rarely, *Yersina pestis* was inhaled directly into the victim's lungs, without contact with a flea, eventually causing suffocation from pneumonic plague.[22]

According to Conrad, tracing the disease according to premodern Muslim sources would always be problematic, given the inability of the authors to understand the disease's biological origin. Thus, they might be able to decipher the buboes, fever and other bodily symptoms, but would not recognise the bacilli as the cause of the disease or rats and fleas as its vectors. Instead, they looked at the plague as a materialistic phenomenon that originated in an elemental-based miasmatic eruption that could be transmitted by corrupted physical elements.

In contrast to Conrad, Michael Dols' account of the 1347–8 outbreak of the Black Death in Mameluke Egypt posits that Islamic societies in general reacted to the plague passively, believing that it was sinful to interfere with the disease as it was God's will. Dols argued that this dogmatic perspective triumphed over the immediate post-1348 accounts like those of Ibn Al-Khatimah (d. 1369) and Al-Khatib, who, like their western European counterparts, shared a miasmatic understanding of the disease.[23]

In Dols' opinion, the Islamic belief that God created a spiritual agent, a genie (*jinn*), who caused the plague to strike, was essential to suppressing miasmatic accounts. This otherworldly view became widely pervasive within a generation of the 1347–8 outbreak, and continued to dominate legal scholars, rulers and the population at large until the modernising reforms of the nineteenth century, which abandoned Islamic law in favour of secular Western-inspired models. To Dols, even later Ottoman accounts like Taşköprüzade's were essential to illustrating how this orthodoxy promoted popular practices, such as the use of 'number magic' and ritual prayer instead of taking physical precautions, like fleeing, or fumigation or other medical remedies. The result, in his view, was the overall decline of the Mamlukes, the Ottomans and other Islamic societies – a key contrast to the West, where views on plague transmission led to extended debate, and the continuing push for reform. He even goes so far as to claim that Western religious treatises on plague, which argued that the disease was God's punishment for sin, was a motivation for moral reform; yet another sign of the Europeans' activist approach towards natural disaster. In his opinion, this activist drive for reform was fundamental to the Western conquest of the disease, progress which culminated in the discovery that the plague was, in fact, caused by *Yersina pestis*.[24]

Heath Lowry's recent article on the plague in the Ottoman Empire in the fifteenth and sixteenth centuries largely confirms Dols' views. Lowry seconds the notion that Islamic societies, particularly the 'core Arabic lands', were dominated by a fatalistic view of Islam that persisted in the succeeding centuries. To Lowry, the Ottomans were an exception to this rule from Osman's founding of the empire in 1300 until Sultan Selim's incorporation of these lands in the wake of the Battle of Çaldıran in 1517. Until this time, 'practical' rulers like Mehmed II, known as 'the Conqueror' of Constantinople in 1453, took activist measures, such as seizing the strategic island of Lemnos – the source of 'Lemnian earth', a popular ingredient in plague medicines – as well as continually repopulating his new capital after it was devastated by the disease.[25] After 1517, however, the Ottomans embraced orthodox Islam and abandoned an activist approach:

> One might well query what, if any, preventive measures did the Ottomans [post-1517] come up with in an attempt to thwart the periodic ravages caused by the plague? The answer is: none whatsoever. It was only in the 1830s that they finally adopted a quarantine regime, a practice which had been in place throughout Western Europe for over 200 years.[26]

Lowry bases these conclusions, like Dols before him, on narrative literature, particularly fifteenth-century Byzantine chroniclers and sixteenth-century Western traveller literature and diplomatic accounts.[27] They coincide with the general claim that the Ottoman Empire, considered by most of its European neighbours to be the gravest threat to Christendom from Mehmed's conquest of Constantinople until Suleyman the Magnificent's siege of Vienna in 1528, had entered a period of stagnation, military defeat, socioeconomic decay and gradual dismemberment that would characterise its history until its ultimate dissolution in 1923.[28]

The most influential work on Ottoman plague during the eighteenth and nineteenth centuries, Panzac's *Le Peste dans l'Empire Ottoman* (1985), almost entirely fits within the historiographical framework that Dols and Lowry have laid out. Panzac argues, on the basis of extensive French and British consular records and traveller accounts, that the Ottomans adopted the maritime quarantine only after extensive European pressure to do so. This European influence was felt in both diplomatic and medical circles. The Europeans, particularly the Habsburgs and the French, apparently suggested both maritime and domestic quarantine in order to combat plague and cholera, a newly emerging epidemic menace in the 1830s. European-trained doctors and newly available published European medical literature popularised quarantine among Ottoman reformers.[29] Panzac concludes that, regardless of Ottoman hesitations, the empire's adoption of the maritime quarantine in 1838 led to the end of this state's dubious distinction as the 'sanctuary of plague'.[30]

Two key works that have explicitly dealt with the critical question of how early nineteenth-century Islamic governments implemented maritime quarantine reform are LaVerne Kuhnke's *Lives at Risk: Public Health in Nineteenth-century Egypt* (1990) and Nancy Gallagher's *Medicine and Power in Tunisia, 1780–1900* (1983).[31] Kuhnke's work illustrates that it was Muhammed Ali, and not the British or French ambassador to Cairo, who initially implemented the maritime quarantine, and, at the same time, the Egyptian Academy of Medicine. These indeed, were key institutions in Muhammad Ali's grand projects of modernisation.[32] The Ottoman sultan Mahmud II, who carried out a similar modernisation programme and implemented the maritime quarantine in Istanbul some seven years after Muhammed Ali's foundation of one in Alexandria, very likely followed the same pattern. Just as Muhammed Ali hired foreign medical experts like Clot, so too Mahmud II employed the Frenchman Sade de Galliere, the Viennese Karl Ambroso Bernard, and the Austrian Anton Lago to help implement the medical reforms.[33] Kuhnke does not discount the fact that the Egyptian medical school, like its Ottoman counterpart, trained new generations of native-born graduates to continue the medical reforms. They may have initially been trained in French, but the language of instruction quickly shifted to Arabic in Cairo and Ottoman Turkish in Istanbul. Despite the gradual decline of these institutions after both the Egyptian and Ottoman governments faced European financial and diplomatic pressure, Kuhnke's findings lead us to believe that the maritime quarantine reform might have been an example of Western-inspired reform. However, the Egyptian maritime quarantine was part of a project of native-led state formation fundamentally distinct from colonial-imposed Westernisation.[34]

Gallagher's work alludes to a similar situation in Tunisia, where the local governor Hamuda Bey (1782–1814) initiated a maritime quarantine in 1784–5. Interestingly, Hamuda Bey launched the quarantine with a host of other measures that restricted French influence over Tunisian exports and imports, all in the name of public health. These mercantilist policies met firm resistance by the French, who publicly protested them by 1828 to Husayn Bey (1824–35), one of Hamuda Bey's successors.[35] While Gallagher, like Kuhnke and Panzac, documents her study with western European language sources, she also makes a serious effort to include relevant Arabic primary source materials, such as Husayn Bey's response to the French protest in 1828, that speak to the issue of quarantines as part of a nativist response to colonial intervention.[36]

This book has benefited tremendously from this historiographical debate, beginning with Conrad's arguments that there was no prevalent dogmatic attitude towards plague among Muslims and that one needs to look at the particular circumstances of each author. Dols' counter-argument that Muslim plague treatises almost universally favoured a fatalistic view has justified the tendency to examine Western travellers, diplomats, politicians and physicians as the primary historical sources about outbreaks in the region.

However, as Gallagher has shown, the most engaging sources were often written by Muslim medical thinkers and statesmen, who hoped to use quarantines and other preventative measures as part of a countrywide policy of modernisation. Unsurprisingly, these reformers would often run into opposition by their western European counterparts, who were frequently attempting to dominate the politics and economy of the region. The common European refrain that the Muslim reformers failed to grasp a truly scientific understanding of the disease often revealed a political subcontext that begs further explanation.[37]

This book seeks to contribute to this scholarship by first looking at the history of plague in the Ottoman Empire prior to 1838 and exploring its relevance to the quarantine reform movement. Chapter 2, 'Conceptualising Plague in Ottoman Islamic Thought', examines how Hamdan's religious justification for the 1838 reform related to prior Islamic thinkers. Hamdan's arguments and the opposition to them were also similar to religious debates on plague and public health in seventeenth- and eighteenth-century England. Chapter 3 'Plague and Ottoman Medical Thought', compares Ottoman medical conceptions of plague with that of Europe. The chapter explores the ties between England, which developed the quarantine in the late sixteenth and seventeenth centuries, and the Ottoman Empire, which did not pursue similar efforts. Chapter 4, 'Magic and Plague in the Ottoman Empire', looks at the continued Ottoman practice of religious ritual and magic to combat plague in contrast to early modern Europeans – particularly the English – whose press culture and religious wars led to increasing repression of individualistic mystical beliefs that defied centralising authority.

The next chapters are dedicated to describing how quarantine reform affected the Ottoman history of plague from 1838 until the end of the empire. Chapter 5, 'Hamdan Bin El-Merhum Osman and the Ottoman Plague Reforms', deals specifically with Hamdan's efforts to establish the quarantine, and contrasts his views to that of British and American writers with regard to sanitary policing. Chapter 6, 'Plague and Quarantines in the Colonial Era', highlights the continuing struggle between the Ottoman authorities, who maintained Hamdan's vision for the quarantine, with that of the British and French, who fundamentally reformulated their conception of plague and the medical institutions connected with them. Chapter 7, 'Plague, Sanitary Administration and the End of Empire', details İzzeddin's final gambit of accepting European social disciplinary methods as part of quarantine reform, underlining how his alienation of the Bedouin of the Hijaz and the Shia of southern Iraq led in part to the disintegration of the Sultanate. Chapter 8, 'Towards a New Understanding of Plague and Quarantines in the Ottoman Empire', wraps up the book with a concluding analysis of the legacy of the quarantine reform movement – Istanbul's maritime quarantine – evident in Golden Horn facilities to the present day.

NOTES

1. Ekmelleddin İhsanoğlu *et al.*, *Osmanlı Tibbi Bilimler Literatürü Tarihi*, vol. 4, pp. 97–8; İdris-i Bitlisi, *Hısn ül-veba: Terceme-i risalet ül-veba*, fols 27B–8A; İlyas bin Abram Al-Yahudi, *Micennetü't-Ta'un ve'l-Veba*; Anton Lago, *Risale-i Karantina*.
2. John Howard, *An Account of the Principal Lazarettos in Europe; with Various Papers Relative to the Plague*; Richard Mead, *A Short Discourse Concerning Pestilential Contagion, or the Plague, with the Methods to be Used to Prevent it*; Richard Mead, *A Discourse on the Plague*; Sir James Porter, *Observations on the Religion, Law, Government, and Manners of the Turks. The Second Edition, Corrected and Enlarged by the Author. To which is*; Patrick Russell, *A Treatise of the Plague: Containing an Historical Journal, and Medical Account, of the Plague, at Aleppo, in the Years 1760, 1761, and 1762.*
3. Anonymous, *The Plague as It Affects England from Official and Other Sources*; Gavin Milroy, *Quarantine and the Plague: Being a Summary of a Report on these Subjects Recently Addressed to the Academy of Medicine in France: With Introductory Observations, Extracts from Parliamentary Correspondence and Notes.*
4. Hamdan Bin Al-Merhum Osman Hoca, *Tercüme-i İthaf el-Munassıfın ve'l-Üdeba bi Mabahit el-İhtiraz'an el-Veba.*
5. Manfred Ulmann, *Islamic Medicine*, p. 94.
6. Ahmed bin Halil er-Rumi, *Risale fi İlmi Tılsım ve Def'i''t-Taun*; Mehmed Süreyya, *Sicill-i Osmanī*, pp. 184–5.
7. Hamdan, *Tercüme-i İthaf*, fols 55B–6A; Kasım İzzeddin, *Hicaz'da Teşkilat ve Islahat-ı Sıhhiye ve 1330 Senesi Hacc-ı Şerifi, Hicaz Sıhhiye İdaresi, Senevi Raporu*, p. 56; Ahmed Midhat, 'Devlet-i Aliyye-i Osmâniye'de Karantina Yani Usûl-I Tahaffuzun Târihçesi', pp. 89–119; Besim Ömer, 'Veba-Ta'un', pp. 218–21, 226–37.
8. Hamdan, *Tercüme-i İthaf*, fols 39B, 45B–6A, 56B–7A, 64B–5A.
9. Anonymous, *Plague*; Milroy, *Quarantine and the Plague.*
10. Kasım İzzeddin, *Hicaz'da Teşkilat ve Islahat-ı Sıhhiye ve 1329 Senesi Hacc-ı Şerifi, Hicaz Sıhhiye İdaresi, Senevi Raporu*, pp. 6–14; Kasım İzzeddin, *Hicaz'da Teşkilat (1330)*, pp. 51–64.
11. İhsanoğlu, *Osmanlı Tibbi Bilimler Literatürü Tarihi*, pp. 972–7.
12. Osman Şevki Uludağ, 'Son Kapitülasyonlardan biri Karantina', pp. 465–7.
13. Lawrence I. Conrad, 'The Plague in the Early Medieval Near East'.
14. Conrad, 'Plague', p. 137.
15. Lawrence I. Conrad, 'A Ninth-century Muslim Scholar's Discussion of Contagion', pp. 166–8, 172.
16. Conrad, 'Plague', p. 459.
17. Conrad, 'Plague', p. 172.
18. Conrad, 'Contagion', p. 177.
19. Conrad, 'Plague', p. 167.
20. Joseph P. Byrne, *The Black Death*, pp. 16–19.
21. Byrne, *The Black Death*, p. 19.

22. Byrne, *The Black Death*, pp. 19–20.
23. Michael Dols, *The Black Death in the Middle East*, pp. 92–4.
24. Dols, *The Black Death in the Middle East*, pp. 284–302.
25. Heath Lowry, 'Pushing the Stone Uphill? The Impact of Bubonic Plague on Ottoman Urban Society in the Fifteenth and Sixteenth Centuries', p. 104.
26. Lowry, 'Pushing the Stone Uphill?', p. 127.
27. Lowry, 'Pushing the Stone Uphill?', pp. 98–9, 125–8.
28. Halil İnalcık, with Donald Quataert, *An Economic and Social History of the Ottoman Empire, 1300–1914*, pp. 400–7; Bernard Lewis, *The Muslim Discovery of Europe*, pp. 33–45; Bernard Lewis, *What Went Wrong? Western Impact and Middle Eastern Response*, pp. 7–17.
29. Daniel Panzac, *La Peste dans l'Empire Ottoman, 1700–1850*, pp. 333–8.
30. Panzac cites Nöel Biraben's conclusions on this matter, pp. 11–13.
31. Laverne Kuhnke, *Lives at Risk: Public Health in Nineteenth-century Egypt*, pp. 49–110; Nancy Gallagher, *Medicine and Power in Tunisia, 1780–1900*, pp. 405, 52–3, 59–60, 98, 106.
32. Kuhnke, *Lives at Risk*, pp. 33–48.
33. Niyazi Berkes, *The Development of Secularism in Turkey*, pp. 112–13; Osman Şevki Uludağ, 'Son Kapitülasyonlardan Biri Karantina', p. 447.
34. Kuhnke, *Lives at Risk*, pp. 51–7.
35. Gallagher, *Medicine and Power in Tunisia*, pp. 24–32.
36. Gallagher, *Medicine and Power in Tunisia*, p. 106.
37. Timothy Mitchell's *Rule of Experts: Egypt, Techno-Politics, Modernity* has looked at the legacy of colonialism and native reaction in public health policy in Egypt from the 1940s until today.

CHAPTER

2

CONCEPTUALISING PLAGUE IN OTTOMAN ISLAMIC THOUGHT

INTRODUCTION

Religious debates on plague and the measures to take against it were of utmost importance in the Ottoman Empire until the 1838 quarantine reforms. Osman bin Süleyman Penah (d. 1817), a prominent medical official during the reign of Selim III (1789–1807) and an opponent of quarantine, understood that the best way to prevent the reform was to undermine its religious legitimacy. The Ottomans, the premier Islamic state from their conquest of Mecca in 1517 until the dissolution of the Empire in 1923, were vulnerable to his criticism that the plague was a blessing from God, to which all Muslims should resign themselves. Selim III was deposed within three years of Osman's pamphlet on the subject; and the rebels successfully gained popular legitimacy by accusing the ruler of abandoning his faith by pursuing modernising reforms.[1]

Yet Osman's dogmatic argument that any precaution against the plague and other epidemic diseases was a betrayal of the Muslims' trust in God's fate (*tevekkül*) had limited currency among Ottoman plague treatise writers. The majority of authors countered this fatalist position by noting that taking precautions fulfilled God's obligation on people to take the initiative in dealing with worldly trials and tribulations. The first such advocates of individual action (*kaza*) in the Ottoman literature on plague, such as İdris-i Bitlisi, an Ottoman statesman from the turn of the sixteenth century, and Isameddin Ahmed bin Mustafa Taşköprüzade, a prominent mid-sixteenth-century Ottoman judge and scholar, focused more on individual reactions to plague; namely, in the form of seeking medical treatment or attempting to flee a plague-infested area.[2] Later the early nineteenth-century reformer Hamdan Bin El-Merhum Osman Hoca would push for broader public health policy measures, such as definitively defining plague as a materially infectious disease and proposing that the Ottomans implement a quarantine to protect their subjects.[3]

The views of these authors do not form a consensus. The debate on whether Islamic law sanctioned material measures against plague continued up until quarantine was implemented in 1838. What this chapter will argue, however, is that the proponents of proactive measures were able to create a sufficient argument for Hamdan's implementation of quarantine in 1838. Hamdan benefited greatly from the efforts of earlier authors, such as Ebussuud Efendi, the chief religious official in the Ottoman Empire from 1545 to 1574, who sanctioned fleeing as a method of preventing plague deaths as permissible under Islamic law.[4] My findings illustrate that Hamdan and earlier advocates of proactive measures were able to navigate Islamic legal sources, namely, the Quran, Islam's holy book, the sayings of the Prophet Muhammad (*hadis*) and the earlier experiences of the Muslim community to justify reform.

This trend towards reform was not unique to an Ottoman Islamic context and compared with even highly developed western European states, such as England. Here, too, religious dogmatists, this time Protestant Christians, opposed medical reforms like flight and quarantine, and denied that God sanctioned individual and state attempts to overcome epidemic disease. English revisionists also made the case for reform, mindful of a possible public backlash. This chapter, towards the conclusion, will reference such debates to view the Ottoman case in a greater comparative context.

By focusing on questions of fate as opposed to individual actions, the legitimacy of the medical profession, the natural transmission of plague, fleeing plague-infested areas, and the civic duty to protect the Muslim community, the following chapter will show that Ottoman Islamic writers from the fourteenth century onwards, like their English counterparts, generally responded to plague and other issues of human suffering by carefully balancing the needs of faith, namely, the belief that diseases and humans alike were God's creation, and the sanction of human reason's attempts to overcome suffering.

FATE AND INDIVIDUAL ACTION

Ottoman scholars most often framed their discussion of plague around the question of how should humans respond to the suffering caused by the disease if God determines everything? One such answer, seen by the dogmatic Osman, was that God's omnipotence precludes all individual action. He cited a *hadis* where a Bedouin with a herd of sickening camels and sheep said to the Prophet Muhammad: 'The camels are sitting on the sand and passing on a disease called mange (*carrab*) to the sheep.' Muhammad then asked: 'Who got the sickness first? How did the camel get mange?' Osman's conclusion was that 'God imparted the disease to each of the animals' rather than the disease transmitting itself from one animal to another. To him, the fact that the victims in this case were animals and not humans made no difference. God, in his view, thus acts without any intermediary, human or otherwise. Anyone who believed otherwise and/or took precautions cast his own faith in doubt. To him, such beliefs or actions led to the delusion that humans could act like God.

For Osman, a Muslim's only proper response was to resign him- or herself to fate (*tevekkül*), believing that God has extended His blessing if he or his family are struck by plague. If the afflicted was a pious Muslim, then he or she had nothing to fear, since plague was in fact 'a blessing and a martyrdom' in that it dispatched the believer to heaven. Conversely, if a non-Muslim died from plague, it would be a torment, since he or she would be sent to hell. Osman cited the *hadis* where Muhammad stated:[5]

> plague (*taun*) is both God's punishment and blessing. If you are in a place where the plague strikes, you should stay and wait patiently. Nothing will happen to you except God's will. God will give you the same place as a martyr.

Osman further posited that plague was, in fact, the equivalent of holy war. He cites another *hadis* where Muhammad prayed: 'Oh God, please let my people (*ümmet*) die for you in war or in plague (*taun*)! They should die by a thrust (*ta'n*) of the enemies of religion or of *taun*. That way they may become martyrs.' Here he noted that linguistically the Arabic terms for thrust (*ta'n*) and plague (*taun*), or 'one who has been pierced' are variants of the same root. At another point, Osman quoted Ebussuud Efendi, the greatest Ottoman Islamic jurist of the sixteenth century, who in a legal advisory (*fetva*) was asked if martyrs of battle and of plague (*taun*) were equal to each other. Ebussuud repeated (Imam) Ahmad bin Hasan's finding that martyrs from plague and war had the same type of wounds, even down to the scent of their blood. Osman then pointed out that Muslim scholars (*fukaha*) and traditionalists (*muhaddisin*) approved of the ruling.[6] Thus, Osman inferred that the pious Muslim should enthusiastically embrace plague in the same way as he was called upon to fight Islam's enemies.

Others supplemented such arguments by claiming that God punished sinners with plague. For instance, Bitlisi alluded to God in the Quran punishing the Pharoah and the Egyptians for keeping Moses and his people as slaves (Surah 7: 133): 'So We sent plagues unto them: wholesale death, locusts, lice, frogs and blood: signs openly self-explained: but they were steeped in arrogance, a people given to sin.' Hamdan similarly pointed out that Ömer bin Elasin's statement that plague resembled 'a fire that spread through the mountains' was 'a sign of God's punishment'. Osman concurred, stating that God's punishment would be tantamount to defying His will.[7]

Such dogmatic conclusions about plague were also fairly common among Muslim thinkers. To Michael Dols, Ibn Hajar Al-Asqalani (d. 1449) was an exemplary of 'Orthodox Islamic' beliefs that only God can cause plague, that death from plague was 'a blessing and a martyrdom' for Muslims and God's punishment for the infidels. Osman's views also echo the tenth-century Asharite school, a widespread reaction throughout the Muslim world to the Mutazilites, an earlier Abbasid rationalist school of theology. The Asharites denied that humans, or nature itself, had any power of causation. Habits of God formulated all events, atomising time and space, and making autonomous natural law impossible.[8]

Certain Ottoman scholars dissented from these fatalistic arguments. Bitlisi, who wrote an extensive defence of his personal choice to avoid plague in Damascus when he was returning to Istanbul from pilgrimage to Mecca, and Hamdan, an exile from Algeria, who came to the Ottoman Empire after openly defying the French occupation of 1830, believed that natural laws of causation had an autonomous place in the cosmos. To Bitlisi, God created natural reactions that no one should deny: 'One who drinks water is satisfied, but one who denies becomes thirsty. Similarly, a person who sees mortal danger, like the outbreak of plague, naturally becomes afraid.' Bitlisi saw such reactions as being in tune with both worldly and divine needs.[9]

Hamdan took Bitlisi's arguments a step further in an extended article on plague in *Takvim-i Vekaye* (The Calendar of Events), the official Ottoman gazette, when in 1838, he wrote a justification for implementing the quarantine system:[10]

> No one in the world can any longer ignore that God established connections between different objects he created, a kind of reciprocal need and dependence on each other. Thus, for instance, hunger is only stopped by feeding; water quenches thirst; sorrow follows a mistake; the salvation of man depends on worshiping the true God and being true to His laws. At the same time, He assigned all inanimate beings appropriate characteristics, such as the stars, minerals, vegetables and numerous species of animals. [For example], fire burns and water quenches thirst. It is true that the Almighty, if He wishes, can suspend the effect of his laws as happened to Ibrahim. However, that is an exception. [In general], these laws are invariable, as needs can only be satisfied by way of analogous means. That is because hunger requires feeding, thirst water, disease medicine.

Here Hamdan claimed that natural causation explained far more than simple individual reaction to stimuli. He posited instead that the natural laws that governed such causes showed a world where the divine played a limited role in earthly events. God's power was superior, but rarely exercised.

Both Bitlisi and Hamdan also argued that human initiative was key to enacting God's will in such a world. For instance, Bitlisi believed that God gave human beings the gift of rational thought in the expectation that they would use these facilities when in danger. A person's choice of responses in this situation ultimately conformed to God's will. If the individual chose properly he or she would have taken the elected path (*ihtiyar-i vacib*). If, however, he or she chose a response counter to the divine will, God's will would nonetheless prevail. Hence, choosing the right path would confirm rather than contradict the idea of resigning oneself to God. Choosing the wrong path would not conform to resignation, but ultimately would be insignificant.[11]

Hamdan, who seconded these notions, claimed that those who argued about God's other-worldly purposes were betraying His will by refusing to deal with material realities. This diversion into fantasy was contrary to true resignation. In his opinion, resignation meant taking precautions and leaving its ultimate impact up to God.[12]

To both Bitlisi and Hamdan, the most imperative of God's commands was to use one's rationality to avoid danger. For example, Bitlisi invoked the Quranic injunction to eat forbidden food if need be (Surah 16: 115): 'He has only forbidden you dead meat, the blood and the flesh of the swine and any food over which the name of other than God has been invoked. But if one is forced by necessity, without wilful disobedience, then God is oft forgiving, most merciful.' Bitlisi believed wholeheartedly that eating forbidden food when one was in danger of starvation was very much akin to a person who was in peril of losing her or his life to plague. Thus, a Muslim could take a measure to save his or her life, even if it was against Islamic tradition.[13] Hamdan similarly stated: 'Take precaution and get ready by any means but do not put yourself in harm's way: God created you and your actions.'[14]

This focus on human initiative paralleled Hamdan's and Bitlisi's reliance upon Muhammad's and his companions' actions to understand and overcome nature. The main message was that mankind needed to control its own fate, a humanistic argument seen among Islamic thinkers. Moreover, adherents of this view believed that humans could not only understand natural logic – the limits of the created – but even comprehend the limits of the Creator and His need for man as an independent actor. The result for the Ottoman revisionists was a secular understanding of the world that complemented the divine.

JUSTIFYING MEDICINE

Osman, however, saw no divine sanction for human efforts to overcome the terrible disease. Instead, Osman believed that only prayer directed at fulfilling God's will was an acceptable response. Here, he cited a *hadis* about Muhammad and his wife, Ayşe, attending to three companions, who came down with a fever shortly after immigrating to Medina. When Ayşe came to visit the sick, her father Ebu Bekir, one of the companions, asked her to recite a verse. The other companions responded similarly. Ayşe, concluding that the verse they had given her made no sense, approached Muhammad to work out what to do. To her, Ebu Bekir and the companions effectively said that 'if God wants, He will show you the right path'. Osman heartily agreed with such sentiments, but disputed the conclusion of the earlier scholar Ebu Harrire, who pointed out that Muhammad then ordered a prayer to dispatch the fever away from Medina. To Osman, Muhammad's prayer was coincidental. Osman claimed that the only time people prayed to escape plague was in 1349. This incident led to denials that the outbreak was anything other than a blessing. He also disputed Al-Asqalani's conclusion that private prayers were permitted. Osman commented that no one prayed when plague broke out later in the second half of the eighteenth century.[15]

Other Ottoman scholars disagreed. Some, like an anonymous eighteenth-century Ottoman writer, believed that prayer and a pious lifestyle were wholly legitimate ways to combat plague. He listed a thirteen-point guide in this regard, saying that a Muslim could get rid of plague by:[16]

> (1) being completely clean; (2) asking for God's forgiveness; (3) gratefully praising God; (4) asking for Muhammad's intercession while praying; (5) eating according to Islamic law (*halal*); (6) not owning questionable property; (7) not desiring to acquire things; (8) having a peaceful heart and clean ideas; (9) having hidden pleasure; (10) avoiding taking refuge in worldly matters; (11) having healthy beliefs; (12) not being [hypocritical]; and (13) having God illuminate one's heart.

This harkens back to earlier fourteenth-century literature on the Prophet's Medicine, which, as Fazlur Rahman mentioned, allowed 'the general educated public easy access to preventive and curative measures'.[17] Ottoman scholars endorsed these measures as a supplemental method of combating plague. Ebussuud, for example, argued that prayers and other good actions, such as being clean, dressing properly, using exulted speech, giving alms to the poor, worshiping God and bearing witness to the faith helped stop plague.[18]

A host of scholars also judged that prayers and other pious activities were permissible. Ghazali argued that prayer against plague was the ideal means to avoid imminent death. Taşköprüzade quoted Süleyman Darafani on the importance of praying against plague, and said that it was more effective on the holiest days and times. Hamdan proclaimed prayers as permissible according to the Hanafi tradition, the dominant judicial denomination of the Ottoman Empire. Such prayers typically begged God to stop the deadly disease. For example, Bitlisi and an anonymous eighteenth-century writer both called out: 'Oh God, You are the protector! Please make the disastrous plague go way!'[19]

Most Ottoman scholars further posited that Islamic law sanctioned medicine as a legitimate means of helping the sick and needy. For instance, Taşköprüzade alluded to a *hadis* from Ebu Harrire where Muhammad was trying to take care of two companions of his who suddenly became sick. Muhammad brought two physicians to see the patients, but who objected to treatment saying that one should trust in God. Muhammad demanded that the physicians give them medication proclaiming that: 'He who created the problem also created the cure.'[20] This *hadis* illustrates that physicians play an important role in bringing about God's will. The general consensus among Ottoman scholars was that physicians had a legitimate role to play within Islamic society. In this regard one anonymous author wrote that 'acting according to physicians' suggestions is not considered taking refuge in worldliness as opposed to God'.[21] Hamdan similarly concluded that the knowledge of medicine was just as legitimate as that of Islamic law.[22]

Hamdan also called for Islamic thinkers to accept that physicians could come up with more effective treatments based on their own experience: 'There is no need to deny things proven by experience.' He went on to conclude that new precautions based on experience were not innovation (*bidat*): medical knowledge was separate from religion and inspiration. Both spiritual and experimental sources were acceptable cures for disease as long as they did not openly contradict the faith.[23]

Muslim thinkers like Hamdan would use such arguments to praise the work of quarantine and public health policy officials, as well as plague doctors, since their pious work was just as necessary to society as that of any imam. It was also an argument that Ottoman reformers would use to justify the state control of a profession that previously worked under the roof of Christian and Islamic pious foundations.

THE NATURAL TRANSMISSION OF DISEASE

Ottoman scholars also thoroughly debated whether plague or other diseases could be transmitted naturally. Osman, the Ottoman dogmatic who did not believe in natural transmission, recalled the *hadis* that 'there is no contagion (*edva*), no augry, and no bird of death'. Citing the interpretation of the Abbasid scholar Imam Turpeşti, Osman claimed that Muhammad's prohibition was definitive. An anonymous Ottoman writer confirmed this *hadis*. Some questioned the context of the *hadis*, however, especially since the statement was directed 'against heathen divination still in use at the time'. There is also a question about translating the term *edva* as 'contagion'. The term most often used for contagion was *sariye*.[24]

Proponents of contagion cited two *hadis*es that testified to the spread of disease among animals. In the first, Muhammad commented about an animal who became sick after drinking water at a well with another sick animal, proclaiming: 'Do not have the sick interact with the healthy!' The second *hadis* is where Muhammad told the Bedouin with the sick camels and sheep to find the camel that first got the disease. Osman protested that contagion did not explain either case since the exact term *sariye* was never used explicitly. Others took a different view. Taşkoprüzade believed that God may have started the disease, but it spread from animal to animal thereafter. He traced his opinion to Imam Turpeşti.[25]

Hamdan added his own insights on rabies (*mümriz*), questioning those scholars who believed that the spread of disease was limited to animals and not to human beings. Although Hamdan readily admitted human superiority, the fact that rabies spread from animals to humans proved that the natural transmission of disease occurred between all God's creatures. He therefore concluded that empirical observation shows that intermingling spreads disease.

Ottoman scholars focused their attention on a list of transmissible diseases that the Abbasid scholar Tabid Ibn Qura (d. 901) passed on to his fellow practitioners of medicine. According to Osman the list included leprosy (*cüzzam*), scabies (*uyuz*), smallpox (*çiçek*), measles (*kızamık*), eye pain (*göz ağrısı*); bad breath (*ağız kokusu*) and a variety of plagues (*emraz-i vebeviye*). The most controversial disease from this list was leprosy. Those who believed in contagion most often quoted Muhammad's saying that 'one should escape from leprosy like you would from a lion'. Hamdan, citing Al-Asqalani, argued that it showed Muhammad's wish that people should avoid harm. Osman countered that Muhammad's directive to leave the leper may have been translated incorrectly. In his mind, Muhammad's directive to leave was most likely due to a cause unrelated to disease, such as going to a more agreeable climate.[26]

Those who questioned the natural transmission of leprosy most often cited the case where the Prophet had a dinner with a leper. Osman argued that his action showed that the disease was not contagious. Hamdan also believed that leprosy was not contagious while the victim lived, but following his or her death it was passed on to another victim. An anonymous Ottoman writer maintained that the question of contagion was irrelevant in the light of Muhammad's charitable action. In his opinion, the moral of the story was that people should take care of the sick regardless of personal danger.[27]

Ottoman scholars also examined plague as a naturally transmissible disease. One such instance is the statement by Ömer bin Al-As (573–664) that 'plague was a fire that spread through the mountains'. Rather than focusing the above-mentioned notion that the spread of plague was a punishment from God, Süleyman Ibn Ahmed Al-Tabarani (873–970) thought that nothing would happen to those who got out of the way of plague. Hamdan concurred with this interpretation, adding that the spread of plague could be explained by natural means.[28]

In addition, Taşköprüzade pointed to a *hadis* about a tribe, who, after complaining to Muhammad about the epidemic, were told to leave since they were likely to catch the disease if they remained in the vicinity. Muhammad warned that 'those who remained close would perish'. Osman disputed that Muhammad was referring to the transmissibility of plague, but, as with leprosy, was referring to possible changes in the weather. Here he hinted at another *hadis* where Muhammad ordered a tribe to change the weather after they had said that they were upset with it.[29]

One may conclude, therefore, that scholars came to no clear consensus over whether diseases like plague were transmissible or not. Islamic legalists like Osman never accepted that Muhammad sanctioned the transmissibility of disease; if Muhammad did, it would have shown the limits of divine power. Nevertheless, the clear majority of Ottoman scholars accepted the counter-argument that diseases were, in part, a natural phenomenon. This left the door open for active precautions against the plague.

ON FLEEING

The most common precaution people took in the Empire to ward off plague was to flee an area once the plague had struck. Osman's late eighteenth-century testimony bears witness to this development:

> Some look outside and inadvertently imagine that this terrible disease spreads. If someone in a household is struck by the plague (*taun*), they decide to flee due to the fear of contagion and they go to another location. Sometimes those who remain are firm, and do proper supplication to God and do not change their location. Consequently, three to four die in their household. People are perplexed as a result of these deaths, and change their location in order to expel the terror. The majority of the population surmises [that the disease] is contagious . . . They prefer changing location and have come to support fleeing out of fear. [30]

This statement verifies that most Ottoman subjects understood plague as a naturally occurring phenomenon that required a physical response; namely, leaving the area.

Ottoman statesmen and thinkers had long condoned such practices, however. Bitlisi's defence of his decision to avoid plague in late fifteenth-century Damascus was followed by legal decisions which permitted fleeing on a broader scale. The mid-sixteenth-century Law Code of Süleyman the Magnificent took up the question of epidemics and whether the public should take steps to avoid the disease:

> What is *taun*? Is it recurring? Is it legal to flee and how should those who have fled be judged? According to the sayings of the Prophet and the Muslim community, plague [*taun*] is a *jinn* which has afflicted the Muslim community with God Almighty's permission. A prior case judged that fleeing is not prohibited. However, it is also right for one to pray for God's mercy.[31]

The Code, implemented on an empire-wide scale, condoned fleeing as a permitted custom among the people. The reference here to the spiritual nature of plague should not be confused with the acknowledgement that the disease was, in part, an earthly phenomenon. Ebussuud Efendi, the author of the Code and the single most influential Islamic jurist of his time, further clarified the urgency of sanctioning fleeing when he was asked 'if according to Islamic law plague breaks out in a village if it was permitted for Muslims, their wives and their children to go to a non-Muslim village'. His answer was that 'it was permitted if they trust in God Almighty'.[32] This opinion indicated that fleeing should be allowed even if it transgressed traditional religious principles; namely, that Muslims should live separately from their non-Muslim counterparts.

Opponents of fleeing – like Osman – had a very difficult time dealing with such legal precedents. Osman could only respond by disputing the authenticity of the statement that 'fleeing from plague was acceptable'. He claimed instead that Ebussuud was really referring to leaving a 'wicked place'. This revised understanding would allow Osman to assert that God was directly responsible for transmitting plague rather than admitting natural transmission as the cause. In other words, fleeing was a response to God's direct spiritual action.[33]

Bitlisi took the opposite tack. To him, plague may have been created by God, but once it appeared on earth it took a natural form that required a physical response, most often fleeing. Fleeing, he believed, was an obligatory act of human reason in the face of deadly danger. Someone who successfully fled from plague thereby demonstrated the superiority of his or her rational choice to one's mere animal-like nature. God pre-ordained such a choice, a step that allowed the chooser to become an instrument of divine will.[34]

Bitlisi, together with Taşköprüzade and Hamdan, justified fleeing using Islamic sources that discussed entering or leaving a plague-infested area. The first of the two main sources to discuss the prohibition on entering a plague-infested area is the previously discussed controversy surrounding Caliph Umar (634–44), and his decision to avoid a plague which had struck Damascus in a place called Amwas in 639.[35]

Ottoman scholars hotly debated the significance of the Amwas incident. On the one hand, Bitlisi, Taşköprüzade and Hamdan argued that Umar's choice not to enter Amwas set a legal precedent that Muslim jurists should obey.[36] On the other, Osman cited Ubaydah's dissent as the real moral of the story, claiming that what Umar did was in fact a grave sin. Osman further asserted that Umar later regretted the decision when he went back with his army to Medina. Umar apparently declared to his companion Kasım bin Muhammad: 'O God, please forgive me for my return from Serag!' Osman thereafter condemned the majority of Islamic thinkers for omitting this part of the story in order to justify the prohibition on entering a plague-infested area.[37]

The second source is the *hadis* where Muhammad declared 'if you hear of plague (*taun*) occurring somewhere, do not go to the place'. This prohibition was cited by numerous Islamic scholars from Abdurrahman bin Awf (d. 652), Abu Muslim Al-Khawlani (d. 684) and Imam Bukhari (810–70) to Bitlisi, Taşköprüzade and Hamdan as the definitive word for those who wished to avoid a plague-infested area. Osman bitterly contested this judgement. He first argued that the *hadis* itself was not properly documented. In this regard, he claimed that Imam Bukhari, the first to record the *hadis*, received the material sixth-hand: Bukhari was told it by Hafs bin Umar, who heard it from Sabe, Sabe from Habib bin Evi, Habib from Ibrahim ibn Saad, Ibrahim from Usama bin Zeyd, and Usama from Saad. He contended that this chain of reporters (*isnad*) was defective, and therefore should not be accepted as a valid saying of Muhammad. However, Osman did not specify who falsified the account, and thus did not provide adequate proof to discount the saying.[38]

Osman then made three further counter-arguments. First, Osman said that even if Muhammad's prohibition on entering a plague-infested area was true, Muhammad must have had an ulterior motive: He was concerned about relatives and friends who would claim their loved one died because they had entered. Such gossip, in Osman's opinion, would only encourage people to give into the temptation to flee death. Second, he claimed that a person who thought that entering a plague-infested area would lead to death was in fact betraying his faith in God's divine providence. Thus, this saying was blasphemy. Third, Osman argued that one could enter a plague-ridden area if one's trust in God was strong. If a person is destined to die, his or her fate would guarantee that person a place in Heaven. If he or she was not struck down by plague it would be an act of God's mercy.[39]

Hamdan also wished to loosen the prohibition on entry, albeit for entirely different reasons. He agreed that the bulk of the population should not be allowed to enter a plague-infested area, but he wished to make an exception for state officials, particularly those who would implement public health measures like a quarantine. He argued that those officials should be allowed into walk into danger in order to protect the Muslim community.[40] This assertion built on Ebussuud's sanction of fleeing and prayer for the common good.

Arguments about prohibiting leaving a plague-infested area rely on two of Muhammad's other sayings. In the first, Muhammad exclaimed: 'Whoever is fleeing from plague (*taun*) is like someone who is fleeing from an enemy on a battlefield. If you are a patient with plague, you are like someone struggling with the enemy.' Muhammad's wife Ayşe apparently added that those who fled plague were like deserters from battle. Critics of fleeing emphasised Ayşe's interpretation, believing that taking precautions was, in effect, abandoning one's duty to struggle (*jihad*). To Osman and others like him, the moral was to abandon precaution and resign one's fate to God.[41]

Supporters of fleeing, namely, Bitlisi and Hamdan, ignored Ayşe's commentary and tried to work their way around the prohibition. They believed instead that Muhammad sanctioned fleeing as a way to 'arm oneself for the holy struggle'. They each cited Ghazali's statement that God predestined both the plague and the prayer meant to repulse it: if plague was a shaft, prayer was its arrow. Hamdan elaborated: 'When you are fighting in war and kill people, it is actually God who kills, not you. When you strike an enemy on the battlefield, it is really God who did it, not you.'[42]

Bitlisi and Hamdan used Ghazali's images to alter the interpretation of the battlefield saying in two fundamental ways. First, they have taken Ghazali's endorsement of prayer to ward off plague as implying that physical precautions like fleeing from plague were equally valid. This is ironic given Ghazali's standing as the great mystic of his age, who spent much of his time critiquing philosophers who argued in favour of experience and innovation. Second, Bitlisi and Hamdan used Ghazali's imagery of spiritual precaution as a weapon to turn Ayşe's 'deserter' into a 'holy warrior'. Bitlisi believed himself to be a perfect example of such a 'holy warrior'. Hamdan argued that it was the Muslim community that could become holy warriors by leaving a plague-infested area. This once again showed his attempt to transform the Ottomans' belief in jihad as a justification for holy war into a legitimisation of society's struggle for a better way of life.[43]

Ottoman supporters of fleeing similarly tried to bend the meaning a second *hadis* where Muhammad warned people 'not to leave a plague-infested area'. Ebussuud attempted to redefine Muhammad's warning as a 'reprehensible' (*mekruh*) rather than a forbidden act (*haram*). He argued that plague was a punishment from God that was not always meant for everyone in the area it struck. Therefore, those who were not the targets of God's wrath should flee the premises. Osman countered Ebussuud's argument by looking at the case of the guilty who likewise tried to flee. Since these people were also targeted for divine punishment, they may well spread the plague to other areas. Hamdan dismissed both of these arguments and believed instead that God would strike those who he had intended without regard to the innocent. Fleeing, like all precautions, 'was a habit whose impact is left to God'.[44]

Hamdan then took another angle by introducing medical experience as a reason to loosen the prohibition on leaving a plague-infested area. He posited that physicians had recently shown that those who left an area immediately after a plague had broken out stood a greater chance of escape if they left immediately. Those who could not go should be left behind.[45]

One may draw a number of conclusions from these extended debates. First, both those who favoured and those who opposed fleeing as a precaution against plague were forced to contradict Muhammad's sayings. Those who supported fleeing may have accepted Muhammad's sayings not to enter a plague-infested area without question. But at the same time they contradicted those of Muhammad's sayings which prohibited people to flee from a plague-infested area. Similarly, opponents of fleeing defended Muhammad's prohibition on leaving an area, but denied prohibitions on entry.

Both sides used arguments about predestination to bolster their opinions. Both sides agreed that plague tested those who were nearby when it struck. To opponents of fleeing like Osman, a Muslim 'passed' the 'test' by not giving in to his fear, and remaining in the vicinity of the plague-infested area. Those who 'failed' gave in to their temptation and fled. In making this decision they gave up their spiritual beliefs in order to save their lives. This would be futile, since God, the direct cause of the disease, would take all He wished.

To proponents of fleeing, the 'test' was using one's reason to avoid harm. To Bitlisi and Hamdan those that 'passed' realised that plague may have been initiated by God, but was in fact a natural phenomenon that acted according to natural laws, including transmission. God expected dutiful Muslims to realise this and respond by fleeing: a physical precaution. There was no spiritual consequence for those who failed, but their natural lives may have been at stakes.

Both sides contradicted these arguments at times. If we take Osman's position,[46] for instance, how could a person who was targeted by God spread the disease to someone who was not? If this was so, would not this mean that plague was spread by natural transmission instead of by divine purpose? Conversely, Ebussuud said that those who were not targeted by God had the right to flee a plague-infested area.[47] This would make no sense if plague was spread simply by divine purpose. He instead implied that plague worked by natural and divine means simultaneously. Similarly, Hamdan's point that precautions were predestined leads one to think that humans could ultimately not understand the rationale God used to organise and interact with the world.[48] Would not recognition of God's inherent superiority lead people to conclude that human rationality was limited? It seems that Hamdan instead laid the foundation for rationalising the sources of faith to justify his own reform programme.

Finally, one wonders why Bitlisi and Hamdan so strongly advocated fleeing as a way of avoiding plague given their personal motives. Bitlisi certainly refused to enter Damascus when he found out it was plague-infested, but he did not 'flee' since he was never there in the first place. Hamdan's idea of quarantine did not technically involve fleeing: those who were caught in a plague-infested area should stay and those who were outside should not enter it. Thus, it is puzzling that Hamdan argued in favour of a person's right to leave an area the plague had struck. The only hesitation Hamdan seems to have had was the need of state officials to enter a plague-infested zone for the good of public health.

Nevertheless, one should highlight a central difference between the proponents and opponents of physical precaution against plague: the proponents actually carried out reforms. Just as Ebussuud legislated fleeing as an option for Ottoman subjects, so, too, Hamdan implemented quarantine as a part of the nineteenth-century *Tanzimat* reforms. Bitlisi and Hamdan faced opposition from some Islamic jurists, but ultimately their ideas won out. Despite Osman's opposition, Hamdan's work was the final word on Islamic law and official measures against plague.

CIVIC DUTY

The last problem that proponents of reform needed to overcome was that of civic duty: if people fled a plague-infested area en masse, who would care for those who were left behind? Even proponents of fleeing, like Bitlisi, Taşköprüzade, Ebussuud and Hamdan, raised doubts. All argued that the poor and the sick would suffer if everyone left them; the dead would not be buried; and strategic places could fall into the hands of the enemy. Moreover, those who fled might truly regret their actions after they heard of the plight of their neighbours and loved ones.[49]

In this sense, Prophetic Medicine, which prescribed charity as a primary component, played a critical role. Ghazali, the advocate of prayer as a means to combat plague, argued strongly that it was the moral duty of Muslims to take care of their own. Hamdan concurred. One could not ignore Muhammad's injunction that Muslims should help each other, that they should take care of the sick, and properly bury their dead. Proponents of fleeing reluctantly agreed. Bitlisi claimed that fleeing was sanctioned only if most stayed behind to take care of the rest. Taşköprüzade stated that one should not flee a plague-infested area if it caused disorder, either in one's household or in the community at large. Ebussuud also hinted at the need of the state to maintain social order.[50]

Some even went so far as to argue that charitable action would also protect someone against plague. Our anonymous eighteenth-century writer claimed that 'those who help plague victims with food and sustenance will be protected' and that one who 'gives alms by meeting the funeral expenses of a plague victim will be saved from the disease'.[51] Here Osman's call for people to simply resign themselves to fate had little resonance. To Hamdan, only a saint could endure such hardship. This lifestyle, however, was not meant for the common people. The moral of the argument was that the response to plague always had to take society's most vulnerable into account. As Ghazali stated: 'You should act properly towards the weak among you' and 'walk at the same pace as the weakest among you'.[52]

The answer to resolving doubts about the needs of the poor was state intervention. Ebussuud pointed out in the mid-sixteenth century that the state would continue to meet society's needs even when people had fled from plague. Hamdan's reform-era quarantine was a far more ideal solution. People did not have to flee, but in the worst case would be confined to their homes in neighbourhoods. Quarantine stations would target travellers, foreigners and merchants far more than common subjects. In time, the Ottomans would come to regard the quarantine system as a mere extension of the welfare state. Nevertheless, Hamdan's quarantine reform helped to convey the powerful understanding that the Muslim community's 'greater jihad' was its internal struggle for a life free of suffering; a key justification for social reform, particularly in the nineteenth century, when the Ottoman Empire had given up any hopes of dominating its European rivals.

Fazlur Rahman pointed out that there is a rich stream of *hadis*es that support social activism, and potentially public health measures such as the quarantine that Hamdan was proposing. At one point Muhammad asked: 'Did you see the one who gives the lie to the faith?' He answered that: 'It is he who maltreats orphans and works little for the feeding of the poor. Woe betide, then, those who pray yet are neglectful of their prayers.' He later stated bluntly that 'When an orphan cries, God's throne shakes' and that 'a person who helps the widows and helpless is waging jihad'.[53]

ENGLISH COMPARISONS

One should consider such discussions on fate and individual action, justifying medicine, the natural transmission of disease, fleeing and civic duty outside a purely Ottoman or Islamic context. For instance, one finds many parallels between the above arguments on fate and individual action among Protestant English religious thinkers from the sixteenth to the eighteenth centuries. One constant line of argument among the English echoed Osman's dogmatic view that God was omnipotent and directly responsible for choosing who contracted and died from the plague. These English dogmatists further posited that God alone was aware of the ultimate causes and purposes behind a plague outbreak. In their eyes, humans could not necessarily understand, for example, what sin a plague victim was being punished for, when God had determined that a person's time on earth was at an end, or if dying from plague was a blessing since a worse fate was in store for the survivors.

Again like Osman, the English dogmatists argued that the worshiper should resign him- or herself to God's fate rather than dwelling on imperfect, finite human logic, or the emotional distress of losing a loved one. The focus for both visions was clearly on God rather than on His prophets or, in the Christian case, Jesus Christ. The English dogmatists, like Islamic thinkers, would cite the example of God punishing the Pharaoh for enslaving Israel by striking down the Egyptians with plagues, particularly the final one brought by the Angel of Death which killed the first-born male of every family. The Angel, who acted directly on God's orders, may have killed 'innocent' children, but the action served the teleological purpose of saving God's chosen people. Denying God's agency and justice was blasphemy.[54]

These views found a ready audience in England. The majority of printed works on plague are sermons which reflect such lines of argument. The sermons, like the other English literature on plague, were mainly published during plague years (for example, 1625, 1636, 1665 and 1720), when public concern was undoubtedly high. One also sees that the authors of such texts were often dissenting English Puritan Protestants, who differentiated themselves from the state-oriented Anglican Church of England. Unsurprisingly, their criticism of individual action to prevent plague deaths dovetailed with their general condemnation of High Church, pro-quarantine rulers (for example, Charles I and Charles II).[55]

Opposing the English dogmatists were those who maintained that God was purely good, but did not determine all events. These English 'revisionists' admitted that plague was evil in the sense that it caused suffering and death. Plague, like other evils, was the consequence of mankind's fall from grace in the Garden of Eden; an agent that destroyed the flawed, compromised and imperfect.[56]

God had created man in His own image, and, having placed him above all other creatures, gave him the task of using his reason to prevent such human misery. If man, the steward of nature, were to do nothing but resign oneself to God's fate, he would in fact be betraying God's trust. He should instead put his knowledge into practice by following the example of Jesus Christ, the Second Adam, whose example of individual action would pave the way for mankind's rehabilitation. He should bear in mind Jesus' continual healing of the sick, his watching over his followers and the downtrodden, and above all, his self-sacrifice even when he could count on God the Father for divine intervention. This is perhaps best illustrated when Jesus, after being tempted by the Devil to cast himself down from the Temple Mount to be rescued by God, refused, saying that this would be giving into sin by needlessly taking advantage of his divinity.[57]

One sees once again similar discussions on the function of prayer and justifications for medicine in the English literature on the subject. One witnesses, for instance, that English prayer writers also sought to mobilise their worshipers' sense of moral reform in order to combat the disease. This can be seen, at least indirectly, in a 1561 'parody on such nostrums':

> Take a pound of hard penance, and wash it down well with water of your eyes, and let it lie a good while at your heart. Take also of the best fine faith, hope and charity that you can get, a like quantity of all mixed together, your soul even full, and use this confection every day in your life, while the plagues of God reigneth. Then, take both your hands full of good works commanded by God, and keep them close in a clean conscience from the dust of vainglory, and ever as you are able and see necessity to use them. This medicine was found written in an old Bible book and it had been practiced and proven true of many, both men and women.[58]

This ridicule of prayers for spiritual renewal in such times of adversity is also witnessed in modern scholarship's condemnation of such 'Prophetic Medicine' as a denial of the natural world. This strong materialist bias often misses the social importance of beliefs; namely, as a disciplinary tool to maintain order in a time of crisis. One sees this tendency when Charles II's public proclaimed a general fast when the great plague of 1665 broke out in London. One could well imagine a similar call by the sultan when plague broke out in his realms.

Unsurprisingly, English prayers on plague, like those of their Ottoman counterparts, were extremely popular. The contents of these prayers, however, reflect the greater debate between dogmatists and revisionists that we also saw in the Ottoman case. A minority, largely made up of non-Anglican English dissenters, took up Osman's view that the plague was either God's judgement or blessing and should not be avoided. One prayer published in the wake of the 1720 Marseilles outbreak exemplifies this point of view:

> I bow myself, Oh righteous Lord to thy blessed will; and acknowledge this my visitation to be the just reward of my sins; O visit me here, that I may not suffer for them eternally hereafter; and grant, that I may so truly and earnestly repent of them, so meekly submit to thy chastisement, and have such steadfast faith in Christ my Saviour, that through his death and passion I may obtain the remissions of my sins, and everlasting life after death. Amen, merciful Father, Amen.[59]

The majority of the prayer publications, sanctioned by the official Anglican Church, recall the mainline Ottoman supplication for God to stop the plague:

> Have pity upon us miserable sinners, who are now visited with great sickness and mortality; that like as though didst then command then accept of an atonement and didst command the destroying angel to cease from punishing so it may now please the Lord to withdraw us this plague, and grievous sickness, through Jesus Christ Our Lord. Amen.[60]

One other prayer, published in 1793, goes so far as to acknowledge plague as an infectious disease rather than simply a punishment:

> All reason it is, that we offer unto Thee our most sincere and hearty thanks, for mercifully assuaging the grievous and infectious sickness, with which of late we have been so sorely afflicted, and for restoring again the voice of joy and health to our dwellings.[61]

Here context is once again vitally important. The writers of this passage included it in a collection of common prayers at a time when quarantine reformers and their state sponsors sought to broaden their public appeal. One cannot find an identical validation of contagionist reforms in the plague prayers as they predate the Ottoman quarantines reforms of Selim III (1789–1807) and Mahmud II (1808–39).

One also finds that many English plague pamphlet writers justified medical practice in religious terms similar to that of their Ottoman counterparts. Reacting in large measure to claims that 'physicians [were] . . . [of] no value' since they did not understand God as the primary cause of the disease, these English revisionists posited that God sanctified the physician's work:

> Such an inquiry after natural and second causes, is more proper for a man of skill in physick and philosophy, who may now show their love to mankind, if they can trace the intricate workings of this subtle disease, and prescribe suitable remedies to prevent or relieve – for human means must act their part with God's blessing upon them.[62]

This passage reminds us of the fundamental Protestant notion of 'a priesthood of all believers', where every calling was equal before the eyes of God – even those based on secular, experimental knowledge.

There is no major theological discussion about contagion among the English authors. They were more interested in the larger question of whether plague was of natural or divine origin. Those who made the distinction between contagionist and miasmatic causes looked towards experience, prior physicians and philosophical works rather than scriptural justifications. This stands in contrast to Ottoman Muslim authors who debated the issue more extensively, although they largely concurred that the plague was indeed contagious. The only exception among the English religious pamphlets was one by James Balmford in 1625. Balmford cited leprosy as a biblical example of contagion, since it mentions that people tried to avoid 'the unclean'. This he argued should be extrapolated to include plague, since it was proven to be contagious by natural reason and expense.[63]

Nevertheless, it is also interesting to consider Hamdan's remark about rabies passing from animal to humans, as this widened the concept of contagion beyond mankind. This idea largely paralleled early modern English thinkers, who gradually deconstructed the classical Aristotelian dichotomy of humans as rational/spiritual creatures who stood distinct from irrational, non-soul possessing animals in favour of a new understanding that blurred these categories.[64] Hamdan seemed to be taking a similar line of argument with an added implication: how could a disease be a punishment from God if animals, who could not think or sin, were also among its victims? This reasoning led to a more naturalistic view of disease. Contagion as a rational concept had therefore begun to defy both biological and religious divides.

There is a fairly sharp contrast between Ottoman and English religious thinkers with regard to fleeing. Although both English and the Ottomans wrote on the topic largely during the sixteenth century, the English and other European writers almost uniformly condemned the practice as un-Christian, citing in part that it was a spontaneous reaction by a population fearing death. Beza, for example, condemned flight as a betrayal of one's sense of charity, and Jesus' command 'to do unto others as you would have them do unto you'.[65]

Benjamin Newton, an English writer, reacted with a similar argument on the plight of the plague victim:

> How far [will the fear of contagion] drive far from him all assistance, and relief; how, when he most of all stands in need of help, he shall find none that will venture to administer it to him; [he] shall find no ties of humanity, or kindred strong enough to hinder all mankind from abandoning, and flying from him.[66]

One should not conclude that Ottoman justifications of flight necessarily contradicted these views. It should be remembered that Muhammad's and Umar's commands not to enter a plague-ridden area were directed at the community and did not relate to spontaneous actions to avoid plague out of fear. Bitlisi alone cited fear and individual instinct as a justification for his own personal case. The only writers to second this opinion were Ottoman or English treatise writers, who wrote from a purely experience-based, natural perspective that flight was an effective method of avoiding the disease.[67]

Moreover, many English religious thinkers pushed for quarantine reform by positing that God only sanctioned orderly attempts to protect the community. This is very much in line with Muslim arguments emphasising that Muhammad and his successors acted to ensure the welfare of the faithful. There is no mistaking the English writers' reference to Moses instructing the Jewish people to protect themselves from plague in Egypt by painting a sign of faith on their doors when the Angel of Death was about to pass. At least some pastors recognised that the English practice of quarantining the sick in houses marked by a cross followed this example. The early eighteenth-century preacher O. Hughes, for instance, explained that both Moses and the reformers protected private households:

> Enter into thy chambers, and shut the doors about thee. The Hebrew word, which we translate as chambers, signifies the innermost and safest part of any house; and as much as men usually choose such a part to rest in, the word often in scripture is used to denote the bed-chamber. So that here good men are directed to get into the safest and most secret places, and to shut their doors, to make all safe about them.[68]

This statement did not recognise a crucial difference between the Biblical and English practice. Moses' mark was meant to ward off plague, where the English cross was meant to prevent the sick from going outside the house. Ironically enough, the symbol of a cross also took on new, morbid meaning. One could see it as a symbol that Christ paid for the sins of the afflicted or dying. Thus, the government used the popular fear of suffering and death to reinforce their measure.

One also sees many references among the English to reform the nation during times of plague. The English religious writers had a variety of causes, such as the need to unite as a nation to protect their 'unique' religious and political values:

> There is no nation upon earth that has had greater experience of the divine goodness, than we have had. We have long enjoyed the inestimable blessing of a free and legal government, while other nations have groaned under the violence of arbitrary oppressions. We have had the free use of our reason and the Holy Scriptures allowed us, which under other governments, which yet call themselves Christian, have, for many ages together, been persecuted even to death.[69]

Inherent in such statements is the need to distinguish oneself from others. In this case, it was 'papist', 'arbitrary' continental Europe (read: France);[70] in another it would be the so-called fatalistic Ottoman Empire:

> The [Ottoman] public government [makes] . . . no provision to keep this fatal distemper at a distance from their country, nor may private persons withdraw themselves from the impending danger. With a kind of pious gravity, or shall I not rather call it an enthusiastic stupidity? They will ask, can you flee from God? Or hide yourself from His omnipresence? Will He not find you out in your closest retirement? And can He not reach you at the greatest distance? If your time be come, if the determined period of your lives be at hand, it is vain to seek security. Fate is unalterable, and its stroke inevitable. Allow only the principal, and the conclusions are indisputable.[71]

CONCLUSION

Contrary to this mischaracterisation, this chapter has established that most Ottoman religious writers across many centuries were not dogmatic, essentialist Muslims who uniformly denied proactive measures against plague as a natural disease. The only well-known 'dogmatist' to espouse these views was Osman, himself a one-time reformer under Sultan Selim III. Although Osman was often able to draw on the Quran and other Islamic authorities to support his case, Ottoman revisionists were usually in the majority. By 1838 – a time when the new Sultan Mahmud II was intent on modernising the Empire and resisting revolt and colonisation – Hamdan was able to convince a receptive audience of the need to support quarantine and other new medical innovations. Osman's earlier appeal to divine authority alone in opposition to such measures may even be viewed as a desperate attempt to derail the bureaucratic effort by provoking popular outrage against the government. The reformers attention to seeking greater public support seemed to have largely defused such efforts.

This gradual consensus compared well with even the most 'enlightened', 'reform-minded' European countries, such as England. Key English authorities were able to deftly construct religious rationales for quarantine and related medical reforms as they did for other natural sciences from the sixteenth to the eighteenth centuries. The English opposition largely echoed Osman and the Islamic dogmatic objections towards plague – especially with regard to God's omnipotence and their denial of the natural world. Admittedly, there were differences. Osman, like earlier Islamic dogmatists, raised specific objections to contagion, while English dogmatists categorically disputed the natural explanation of disease. Likewise, the Ottoman revisionists until Hamdan debated the merits of flight from plague, where English revisionists instead approved the quarantine even by the late sixteenth century. Yet the degree to which both the Ottomans and English used similar arguments – on the importance of individual and state efforts to combat human suffering by mastering natural medical science – illustrates that these differences cannot fundamentally be explained in religious terms. Both Islam and Christianity provided modernisers with a path towards reform.

NOTES

1. Süreyya, *Sicill-i Osmanī*, p. 1291.
2. Bitlisi, *Hısn ül-veba*; Ebu's-suud Efendi, *Risale-i Ebussuud*; Kemaleddin Taşköprüzade, *Risale fi't-Taun ve'l-Veba*.
3. Hamdan, *Tercüme-i İthaf*.
4. Berkes, *Development of Secularism in Turkey*, p. 113; Mehmet Ertuğrul Düzdağ, *Şeyhülislam Ebussuud Efendi Fetvaları Işığında 16. Asır Türk Hayatı*, p. 93.
5. Sa'deddin Süleyman bin Muhammed Emin Müstakimzade, *Cihazü'l-Macun fi'l-Halas Mine't-Taun*, fol. 49B; Osman, *Tercüme-i İthaf*, fols 8A, 13A–14B.
6. Osman, *Tercüme-i İthaf*, fols 5B, 10A.
7. Bitlisi, *Hısn ül-veba*, fol. 4B; Hamdan, *Tercüme-i İthaf*, fol. 57A; Osman, *Tercüme-i İthaf*, fol. 8A.
8. Dols, *The Black Death in the Middle East*, pp. 110–13; Fazlur Rahman, *Health and Medicine in the Islamic Tradition: Change and Identity*, pp. 15–16.
9. Bitlisi, *Hısn ül-veba*, fols 6B–7A, 13A; Hamdan, *Tercüme-i İthaf*, fol. 39A.
10. Panzac, *La Peste dans l'Empire Ottoman*, pp. 583–4.
11. Bitlisi, *Hısn ül-veba*, fols 10B, 13A–14A, 15A, 38A–41B, 61A–B.
12. Hamdan, *Tercüme-i İthaf*, fol. 55A.
13. Bitlisi, *Hısn ül-veba*, fol. 56A.
14. Hamdan, *Tercüme-i İthaf*, fol. 41B.
15. Osman, *Tercüme-i İthaf*, fols 19B–20A.
16. Müstakimzade, *Cihazü'l-Macun fi'l-Halas Mine't-Taun*, fol. 43A.
17. Rahman, *Health and Medicine in the Islamic Tradition*, pp. 15–16.
18. Düzdağ, *Şeyhülislam Ebussuud Efendi Fetvaları Işığında*, p. 93.

19. Müstakimzade, *Cihazü'l-Macun fi'l-Halas Mine't-Taun*, fol. 39A; Bitlisi, *Hısn ül-veba*, fol. 77A.
20. Taşköprüzade, *Risale fi't-Taun ve'l-Veba*, fols 93B–94A.
21. Müstakimzade, *Cihazü'l-Macun fi'l-Halas Mine't-Taun*, fol. 43B.
22. Hamdan, *Tercüme-i İthaf*, fol. 66A.
23. Hamdan, *Tercüme-i İthaf*, fols 43B, 60B.
24. Osman, *Tercüme-i İthaf*, fols 7A–B, 12B–13A, 15B–17A; Müstakimzade, *Cihazü'l-Macun fi'l-Halas Mine't-Taun*, fol. 48B; Ulmann, p. 87.
25. Osman, *Tercüme-i İthaf*, fols 13A–15B; Taşköprüzade, *Risale fi't-Taun ve'l-Veba*, fols 93A–B.
26. Hamdan, *Tercüme-i İthaf*, fol. 48A; Müstakimzade, *Cihazü'l-Macun fi'l-Halas Mine't-Taun*, fol. 48A; Osman, *Tercüme-i İthaf*, fols 11A–B.
27. Osman, *Tercüme-i İthaf*, fols 11A–B; Hamdan, *Tercüme-i İthaf*, fols 52A, 54A; Müstakimzade, *Cihazü'l-Macun fi'l-Halas Mine't-Taun*, fols 48A–B.
28. Hamdan, *Tercüme-i İthaf*, fols 48A–B, 57A.
29. Osman, *Tercüme-i İthaf*, fols 8B–9A; Taşköprüzade, *Risale fi't-Taun ve'l-Veba*, fols 93A–B.
30. Osman, *Tercüme-i İthaf*, fols 2A–B.
31. Düzdağ, *Şeyhülislam Ebussuud Efendi Fetvaları Işığında*, p. 93.
32. Düzdağ, *Şeyhülislam Ebussuud Efendi Fetvaları Işığında*, p. 93.
33. Osman, *Tercüme-i İthaf*, fol. 17B.
34. Bitlisi, *Hısn ül-veba*, fols 15B, 37B, 41B, 43A, 44B, 45B, 50B, 51B–52A.
35. For more background on the Amwas debate, see Chapter 1, pp. 7–8; Osman, *Tercüme-i İthaf*, fols 7B–8A.
36. Bitlisi, *Hısn ül-veba*, fols 5A, 52A; Hamdan, *Tercüme-i İthaf*, fols 47A–B; Taşköprüzade, *Risale fi't-Taun ve'l-Veba*, fol. 182A.
37. Osman, *Tercüme-i İthaf*, fols 6A, 7B–8A.
38. Hamdan, *Tercüme-i İthaf*, fols 46A, 50A; Müstakimzade, *Cihazü'l-Macun fi'l-Halas Mine't-Taun*, fol. 44A; Osman, *Tercüme-i İthaf*, fol. 6A.
39. Osman, *Tercüme-i İthaf*, fols 6B, 7B.
40. Hamdan, *Tercüme-i İthaf*, fol. 56A.
41. Osman, *Tercüme-i İthaf*, fol. 17A.
42. Hamdan, *Tercüme-i İthaf*, fol. 41B.
43. Bitlisi, *Hısn ül-veba*, fols 45A, 61B–2A; Hamdan, *Tercüme-i İthaf*, fols 50B, 67B.
44. Hamdan, *Tercüme-i İthaf*, fols 56A, 60A.
45. Hamdan, *Tercüme-i İthaf*, fols 50B, 56A, 68A.
46. Osman, *Tercüme-i İthaf*, fols 15B–17A.
47. Taşköprüzade, *Risale fi't-Taun ve'l-Veba*, fols 100A, 182A.
48. Hamdan, *Tercüme-i İthaf*, fol. 40B.
49. Bitlisi, *Hısn ül-veba*, fols 46B–47B; Taşköprüzade, *Risale fi't-Taun ve'l-Veba*, fol. 94A; Hamdan, *Tercüme-i İthaf*, fol. 54B.
50. Bitlisi, *Hısn ül-veba*, fol. 47B; Hamdan, *Tercüme-i İthaf*, fols 47B, 55B; Taşköprüzade, *Risale fi't-Taun ve'l-Veba*, fol. 94A.
51. Müstakimzade, *Cihazü'l-Macun fi'l-Halas Mine't-Taun*, fol. 49A.
52. Hamdan, *Tercüme-i İthaf*, fols 55B, 56A.
53. Rahman, *Health and Medicine in the Islamic Tradition*, pp. 30–1.
54. William Goldwin, *God's Judgments on a Sinful People. A Sermon Preach'd on the 8th*

of December, Being the Fast-Day, Appointed to Implore God's Protection Against the Plague Now in France, p. 13; Obadiah Hughes, *The Good Man's Security in Times of Publick Calamity. A Sermon Preach'd in Maid-Lane, Southwark, on Occasion of the Plague in France*, pp. 3–5.

55. Hughes, *The Good Man's Security in Times of Publick Calamity*, pp. 8–12.
56. Goldwin, *God's Judgments on a Sinful People*, pp. 13–14.
57. James Balmford, *A Short Dialogue Concerning the Plagues Infection Published to Preserue Bloud, through the Blessing of God: Together with a Sorting of all those Verses in the Psalmes which are Noted with the Word Selah to Shew the Complaints, Comforts, Faith, Prayer and Praise of Gods Children*, pp. 22–4.
58. Charles F. Mullett, 'Some neglected aspects of plague medicine in sixteenth-century England', p. 326. Mullett notes that he modernised the spelling of this passage.
59. Anonymous, *Church of Englandman's Companion*, p. 389.
60. Anonymous, *Church of Englandman's Companion*, p. 265.
61. Thomas Morgan, *A Common Prayer-Book, According to the Plan of the Liturgy of the Church of England, with Suitable Services*, p. 154.
62. Goldwin, *God's Judgments on a Sinful People*, pp. 2–3.
63. Balmford, *A Short Dialogue Concerning the Plagues*, pp. 8–13, 33–7.
64. Andrew Roedell, 'The Beasts that Perish: The Problem of Evil and the Contemplation of the Animal Kingdom in English Thought, 1660–1839', pp. 100–57.
65. Théodore de Bèze Beza, *A Learned Treatise of the Plague Wherein the Two Questions, Whether the Plague be Infectious or No, and , Whether and How Farr it May be Shunned of Christians by Going Aside, are Resolved*, pp. 1–8.
66. Benjamin Newton, *Sermons on Several Occasions. In Two Volumes*, pp. 385–6.
67. Al-Yahudi, *Micennetü't-Ta'un ve'l-Veba*, fols 9A–13A; Simon Kellwaye, *A Defensatiue against the Plague: Contayning Two Partes or Treatises: The First, Shewing the Meanes How to Preserue Us from the Dangerous Contagion Thereof: The Second, How to Cure Those that are Infected therewith. Whereunto is Annexed a Short Treatise of the Small Poxe: Shewing How to Gouerne and Helpe those that are Infected Therewith*, pp. 2–3.
68. Hughes, *The Good Man's Security in Times of Publick Calamity*, p. i.
69. Samuel Clarke, *Sermons on Several Subjects and Occasions By Samuel Clarke, . . . In Eight Volumes. Containing One-Hundred and Ninety-One Discourses, Being all those Published in his Life-Time, and those Since his Death, by John Clarke, . . . With a Preface, . . . by Benjamin, now Lord Bishop of Winchester*, p. 145.
70. Another example of British religious chauvinism can be seen in the following condemnation after the 1720 Marseilles outbreak. Benjamin Grosvenor, *Preparation for Death, the Best Preservative against the Plague. Being the Substance of Two Sermons, preach'd at the Merchant's Lecture in Salters-Hall, Jan. Seventeenth, and 31st, 1721*, p. 42.
71. Thomas Moulton, *This is the Myrrour or Glasse of Helth Necessary and Nedefull for Euery Person to Loke in, that wil Kepe their Bodye from the Syckenesse of the Pestilence, and it Sheweth Howe the Planettes do Raygne in Euery Houre of the Daye and Nyghte, with the Natures and Exposicio[n]s of the xii. Sygnes, Deuyded by the xii. Monethes of the Yeare, and Shewed the Remedies for Many Dyuers Infirmities and Dyseases that Hurteth the Bodye of Mann*, p. 40.

CHAPTER

3

PLAGUE AND OTTOMAN MEDICAL THOUGHT

INTRODUCTION

Although both Ottoman and European religious leaders often sanctioned the fight against epidemic diseases from the sixteenth century onwards, the Europeans undoubtedly adopted quarantine long before the Ottomans. Renaissance writers from Boccaccio to Fracastoro wrote of the contagious nature of plague, and a number of Italian city-states established quarantines as early as the fifteenth century to isolate those sick with plague.[1] Other European states – particularly maritime powers like England and France – adopted the institution during the sixteenth to the eighteenth centuries. London's great plague of 1665 and the Marseilles outbreak in 1720 convinced many of the need to more strictly enforce isolation measures in order to protect people from exposure to deadly diseases from overseas. Even expatriate merchant communities from these countries sought to avoid plague in the Ottoman cities of Cairo, Smyrna and Istanbul by quietly implementing their own quarantines there.[2]

Yet the differences between the Ottomans and the European maritime powers were much more subtle than first meets the eye. Ottomans and other Middle Eastern Muslim plague treatise writers from 1347 to 1600 did not fundamentally differ from their western European counterparts. Both Europeans and Muslims often understood plague in contagionist terms and circulated their works in narrow courtly or academic circles. In fact, European and Muslim scholars would often interact in a way that made it hard to differentiate between the two 'civilisations', as they freely borrowed new concepts, experiences and comparative models from each other.

The gap between the European and Ottoman Muslim perceptions of plague only occurred between 1600 and 1800 with the rise of mercantilism and overseas commercial development in north-western Europe. Institutional reforms like quarantine came as a result of a state-led programme of economic development and radical social change, beginning with maritime states such as England. English plague treatise writers in particular participated in this evolving system. One witnesses fundamental changes in both their social context – an emerging commercial print culture – and ideological content – the mercantilist economic values of their works. In short, they would become new willing contributors to a national economic agenda that would justify mercantilist reform in the name of public health.

Strikingly, the Ottomans did not directly respond to the newer European quarantine and mercantilist discourse until after 1800, when plague treatise writers like Hamdan began to call for reform. The Ottoman government simply did not implement a state-led modernisation programme, much less a quarantine. There were comparatively fewer seventeenth- and eighteenth-century Ottoman plague treatise writers than in the sixteenth century, although they too remained limited to courtly and academic circles. Thus, unlike their English colleagues, they did not participate in print culture or reflect new commercial interests. Nevertheless, their differences with mercantilist plague treatise writers were more economic than cultural, as they, like their sixteenth-century predecessors, remained receptive to new ideas and innovations. The Ottomans had a continued commitment to proactive measures directed at protecting health, and had at least a limited discourse with the outside world. Still, European mercantilist success would eventually pressure the Ottomans by exposing them to new commercial and military threats. Commercially, the new mercantilist powers, especially England, would disrupt the Ottoman economy and even threaten its sovereignty in the name of modern, western European public health. Politically, this ideological threat would lead to growing demands for the empire's partition and colonisation.

EARLY MEDICAL CONTRIBUTIONS

Scholars have argued that western Europeans had responded differently to plague than their Muslim counterparts ever since the initial 1347–8 outbreak. The first evidence they point to is Europe's popular reaction to plague as a contagious disease.[3] Boccaccio, who wrote his famous *Decameron* in the immediate aftermath of the Black Death in Florence summed up this attitude:

> What gave more virulence to this plague, was that, by being communicated from the sick to the hale, it spread daily, like fire, when it comes in contact with large

> masses of combustibles. Nor was it caught only by conversing with, or coming near the sick, but even by touching their clothes, or anything that they had touched before.[4]

As a result, people '[avoided] the sick, and everything that had been near them . . . Others . . . in greater numbers left the city, their houses, relations and effects, and fled into the country'. Boccaccio decried these practices as utterly inhumane, since the sick and poor were often left to fend for themselves, without proper care, food and water. He believed that many died needlessly as a result.[5]

Most scholars see the establishment of quarantines in places like Florence and other Italian city-states within a generation of the 1347–8 outbreak as a natural response to these threats to the social order. Containing the disease within restricted areas, such as boats and guarded hospital wards, where plague victims could be isolated but cared for, seemed to resolve the problem.[6]

Most historians of the plague admit, albeit reticently, that early modern medical thinkers generally did not accept such notions. Instead, they, like a number of their Muslim colleagues, came to a different consensus about the plague's causes, preventive measures and cures. In their opinion, plague was originally a corruption of the air that disturbed all creatures' natural humoral balance. Earthquakes, fetid water, rotten corpses, a southerly wind or intemperate weather could all cause the ill-wind to blow, forcing frogs, rats, insects and birds to flee and striking down all who remained. Once a victim breathed in the poisonous air, the heart, the chief organ of the body, would overheat and lead to a mortal fever. The victim would display a variety of other agonising symptoms before death, including headache, light-headedness, sore throat, buboes, coughing up blood, profuse sweating, pain and discolouration on the side, the armpits and the groin.[7]

The medical writers also prescribed uniform preventive measures and recommended specific dietary measures that would strengthen one's humoral balance and the heart, such as figs, dates, raisins, nuts, pomegranates, light white wine and fresh spring water. They prohibited certain foods, such as leguminous vegetables, meat, milk and fish since they were prone to spoil quickly, and were affected to a much greater degree by the corrupt air.[8]

Furthermore, the writers believed that one could prevent plague by changing the environment. They believed, for instance, that those who sought higher ground could avoid plague, since the corrupt air tended to remain in low places. Those who had to stay in affected areas could still burn incense or dry, aromatic wood and herbs. Additionally, people should avoid bathing, as this would open one's pores to the moist, sickly air.

Cures were also aimed at restoring the victim's humoral balance, although the writers conceded that these were desperate measures. They included blood-letting or 'cupping', classical medical ingredients like rose water, vinegar, lemon, Armenian earth and spices like black pepper.[9]

Historians of medicine ironically note that Al-Khatimah and Al-Khatib, both Muslim writers from the Umayyad kingdom of Granada, would be among the first medical thinkers to mention the contagious nature of the disease. Like Boccaccio, both Al-Khatimah and Al-Khatib wrote their works in the immediate aftermath of 1347–8. Al-Khatimah, wrote, for instance, about his own personal encounters with the plague:

> The best which long experience has taught me is that when anyone comes into contact with a sick man, forthwith the same disease seizes him, with the same symptoms; if the first sick man has spit blood, he also spits it; if the former was hoarse, he likewise becomes hoarse; if with the first buboes appeared on the groin, so do like buboes appear in the same place with the other; if with the first a boil arose, there arises with the second in a like boil; also the second sick man carries the sickness on farther. The family suffers in the same way, shows the same symptoms; if the sickness of one member runs a fatal course, the others suffer the same fate; if the sick man is saved, so they also escaped death. In this way on the whole, with slight differences, has it gone in our city.[10]

However, Al-Khatimah would later go on to deny the contagious nature of disease, since he contended that contagion was contrary to Islamic law. Historians cite this reversal as a key point in the history of medicine, as it showed that Muslim religious orthodoxy stifled the development of critical, experimental thought.[11]

Al-Khatib, a friend and close companion to Al-Khatimah, heartedly objected to such restrictions:

> If one asks 'How can you admit the assertion there is infection, when the revealed word denies this?' We answer: that infection exists, [and] is confirmed by experience, research, insight, observation and through constantly recurring accounts. These are the elements of proof. For him who has treated or recognised this case, it cannot remain concealed that mostly the man who has had contact with a patient infected with this disease must die, and that, on the other hand, the man who has had no contact remains healthy. So it is with the appearance of the illness in a house or quarter because of a garment or a vessel; even an earring can destroy him who puts it in his ear, and all the inhabitants of the house.[12]

European writers, beginning with Fracastoro, picked up on these ideas in the sixteenth and seventeenth centuries. Fracastoro argued specifically that 'seeds of contagion' were responsible for the spread of the plague, and not just moist, corrupt air that passed from person to person. Modern authors judged that Fracastoro's prediction that germs were responsible for the spread of disease presaged the end of the Galenic system of thought.

Many scholars also see Fracastoro as an almost revolutionary figure who bridged the gap between popular contagionism and literary elites, and led future generations of medical thinkers to directly participate in formulating quarantines and other related public health policy reforms. They also point to Fracastoro's use of new inventions, such as the printing press, to disseminate his contagionist ideas. These developments, in turn, helped early modern states to extend their social control over the population, and in the process, helped to generate commercial development.[13]

These arguments beg careful reconsideration. First of all, it is not clear what connections Fracastoro had with his quarantinist contemporaries. Fracastoro's works did appear at a time when Italian city-states such as Venice and Florence had quarantines. However, the expansion of the quarantines to urban bureaucracies specifically dedicated to epidemic control, permanent plague hospitals (lazarettos) and cadastral registers of the dead began only some fifty years after his death, at a time when maritime states sought greater economic and social control over their populations. Fracastoro's claims may have been popular among academic circles in northern Italy and southern Germany, but they did not spur debate between quarantine officials and the Italian commercial elites who, facing new expenses and restrictions on their Mediterranean overseas trade, may have opposed them.[14]

Despite these limitations, historians contrast the dynamic growth of contagionist thought with Muslim writers, whom they contend simply ignored Al-Khatimah's and Al-Khatib's initial accounts. At best, Muslim writers restated Galenic maxims about the miasmatic and humoral origins of the plague, and, at worst, followed Al-Khatimah's lead in repressing medical thought in the name of religious dogmatism.[15] Yet to date there has been little serious consideration of what this 'second generation' of Muslim scholars, the bulk of whom were late fifteenth- and sixteenth-century patrons of the Ottoman court, actually wrote about the plague.

There is a remarkable amount of contagionist and innovative thought among these writers, however. For instance, Bitlisi wrote prior to Fracastoro in around 1500 that plague and other diseases were contagious:

> Plague is spread by smelling, touching and seeing. This contagion is similar to what happens with rabies among dogs and other animals. With rabies, dogs

> spread the disease by biting others. As I have seen by experience, rabies also spread just by touching and breathing.[16]

This passage is especially significant as Bitlisi grounded his assertion in his own experience, not just what he read. This cuts against the argument that Muslim authors either repeated Galenic maxims or rejected scientific innovation.

Other authors supported their own observations with attributions to earlier Muslim writers. Bitlisi, an anonymous seventeenth-century Ottoman writer and Osman, a late eighteenth-century anti-contagionist critic, claimed that Muslim doctors long considered plague to be one of the great contagious diseases, a status shared with leprosy, mange, fetid breath, measles and smallpox. Similarly, Al-Yahudi, a late fifteenth-century Jewish convert to Islam who fled to the Ottoman court, asserted that Avicenna personally witnessed the contagious nature of plague. He also said that 'Ibn Rüshd [Avveroes] of Cordoba mentions that a person who isolates himself can avoid plague'. This raises the curious argument that even key twelfth-century Islamic thinkers could presage the idea of a quarantine some two hundred years before the Black Death. Perhaps Al-Yahudi sought to cover his own personal arguments – like his warning 'not go in crowded districts' – with earlier renowned authorities so that his recommendations would be accepted within literary Islamic traditions.[17]

Most early modern Ottoman treatise writers advocated fleeing as a measure to avoid plague. As seen in Chapter 2, Bitlisi's own work is an extended Islamic legal justification of his own flight from a plague outbreak in Damascus and parts of Anatolia when he was returning from a pilgrimage from Mecca.[18] Al-Yahudi scrupulously avoided such legal arguments, and accepted the 'most experienced Christian physicians' suggestion to flee from a plague infested area' since 'even the birds and animals cannot endure'.

Al-Yahudi and the other early modern Ottoman writers made some provocative prescriptions as cures for the plague. Al-Yahudi stated a number of times that wine was a good remedy, without mentioning that Islamic jurists almost universally condemned consuming alcohol, and wine in particular. The seventeenth-century anonymous author made a similar suggestion. Al-Yahudi also mentioned that Avicenna prescribed plague victims to drink a Venetian treacle, a complex concoction that also included alcohol and snake blood, both prohibited by Islamic law. Al-Yahudi disagreed, but only because he did not see it as effective in practice.[19]

Other authors also made surprising prescriptions. An anonymous seventeenth-century prescription collection included opium and sulphuric acid among its ingredients, alongside the more traditional garlic, onion, vinegar and rose water.[20] Such chemicals were hardly the rule for 'traditional' Galenic medicine. Moreover, Bitlisi went so far as to suggest the use of quicksilver, a chemical that came into vogue in Europe at roughly the same time that he wrote his work. Bitlisi mentioned that he not only used the drug for plague during an outbreak in Diyarbekir, but also even earlier when the first syphilis pandemic broke out in Europe in 1494:

> It [syphilis] was not heard of by our ancestors or from earlier philosophers. The above-mentioned disease appeared in European lands (*efrenc*). Since Anatolia is close to Europe, it spread from the latter to the Arab, Persian, Indian and Chinese lands. It was called '*ceb-i efrenc*' due to its origin. It is now called '*frangi*'. Many people died among the Muslims. The medication which was prescribed during this outbreak was unknown previously to physicians and philosophers and was not cited in medical books. The medication included melted quicksilver (*erbak-i mahlul*). A number of another chemicals and elements are mixed with melted quicksilver to produce the medication. I even used this drug for four months and was cured because of it.[21]

Bitlisi's advocacy of chemical prescriptions was freely borrowed from his European contemporaries and not from previous authorities.[22]

The first modern Muslim reformists were often dismissive of Bitlisi and the early Ottoman plague writers, claiming that the audience and impact of this literature was minimal. Such views were very important, as they justified the claims of later historians that the Ottomans did nothing substantial about plague and other epidemic diseases until the reforms of the 1830s. Sultan Mahmud II's eloquently expressed this argument when he gave his inaugural address for the empire's first European-style medical school in 1835:

> It is true that many books were written among us [Muslims] on medical sciences and that the Europeans even learned many things by translating these books into their own languages. The books were written in Arabic, however, and, as they ceased to be objects of interest and care in the Muslim schools for many years and as the number of men who knew them decreased, they became obsolete. To go back to these works now and plunge into their study in order to translate the science of medicine into our own language, Turkish, would be a painstaking job actually requiring many years.[23]

Here Mahmud II makes the assertion that earlier Ottoman medical thinkers, plague treatise writers included, in general had outdated ideas and wrote in classical Arabic, supposedly a language which was foreign to Ottoman Turks and others of the empire's ethnicities. This statement also implies that the Ottomans suffered from a lack of print culture and other technological developments that widened the public and scientific reception to new medical ideas.

But one should weigh his statements carefully. Although Bitlisi, Taşköprüzade and Al-Yahudi's works were still in circulation in the early nineteenth century, as is evident from a rise in manuscripts on the topic during Mahmud II's reign, it is ironic that a number of these new manuscripts were in fact translations of texts from Arabic to Ottoman Turkish. These translators included Ahmed Kürkzade, a prominent early nineteenth-century Ottoman notable from Istanbul, and Muhammad Salih, a major figure within the Nakşibandi *tarikat* from eastern Turkey and an important player in the imperial political scene after Mahmud II had deposed the Janissaries and the rival Bektaşi *tarikat*. Both translators believed that their efforts were important to ongoing discussions about plague and other epidemic diseases, such as cholera, which had broken out at roughly the same time period.[24] If Mahmud II saw these works as a waste of time and effort, a number of other participants in Ottoman literary culture fundamentally disagreed.

Nevertheless, one should not underestimate the impact Bitlisi, Taşköprüzade, Al-Yahudi and the other early modern Ottoman authors had on audiences from the late fifteenth to the mid-seventeenth centuries. They were indeed aimed at a variety of circles, including religious and urban elites, Ottoman statesman and court circles. Many in this audience were fluent in classical Arabic: a legal and ecclesiastical language used in many ways like Latin in much of central and western Europe. Moreover, a considerable number of readers who saw the works in collections in Istanbul and other regional cities (for example, Damascus, Cairo and Salonika), doubtless passed on what they read to third parties. They could have conceivably read them to others or summarised them orally. They could have conveyed these ideas in an institutional setting, such as an Islamic school (*medrese* or *mekteb*), a local judge's court, at a local mosque or pious foundation, at market or even on the street. Some ideas may even have penetrated emerging coffee houses, where minstrels could talk of some materials, like Bitlisi's adventures, as a traveller's tale. Certainly, the works did not have the benefit of a printing press, but such a medium did not begin to have a full impact on medical and scientific developments until the overseas commercial developments of the mid-seventeenth century.[25]

One should also note that a number of the key plague treatises – such as Taşköprüzade's and two anonymous seventeenth-century works – were translated at that time into Ottoman Turkish by highly respected members of the literary elite, such as Ebussuud Efendi, the single most influential Ottoman Islamic jurist of the sixteenth century, and Abdulgani Efendi, a well-known seventeenth-century religious figure. Although much of the early modern literature on plague remained in Arabic, their translations helped to sow the seeds of Ottoman literary culture.[26] This mixture of vernacular with ecclesiastic languages is a familiar one, considering that a similar discourse was witnessed in Europe at that time.[27]

In retrospect, one may first conclude that Muslim treatise writers, and the Ottomans in particular, exchanged new ideas on all aspects of the plague from the Black Death of 1347–8 until the late sixteenth century. In this regard there was no major difference between European and Muslim authors. The question of whether Muslims and Europeans had differing popular reactions is still open, but the frequent suggestions of contagion, fleeing and even Al-Yahudi's hint that isolation was justified may be evidence of similarity on many fronts. One can say with relative certainty only that historians have generally overstated the case that Europeans alone reacted to plague with measures based on experience and scientific observation.

It is also difficult to make geographic or comparative notions about the dissemination of knowledge and the origins of disease. One frequent thread in the history of knowledge maintains that any innovation in Muslim civilisations was due to the 'importation' of that idea from Europe. Edward Gibbon, for example, goes so far as to claim that the Abbassid translators of ancient Greek texts into Arabic were Christian Greeks and that the Arabs themselves distained learning a heathen tongue.[28] Yet such arguments cannot adequately explain how other writers, like Bitlisi, could succeed in introducing new medical ideas, since he was not of European origin and did not even travel to non-Muslim lands. How could a Muslim so freely exchange thoughts on combating plague that were in vogue in Europe at the same time, if there was not an intricate and ongoing cultural, social and intellectual exchange between the two cultures?

Instead, the focus should be on the multicultural experience of many of the plague treatise writers. Al-Yahudi, the Sephardic Jewish refugee, found his counterpart in Bitlisi, who likewise fled as a Sunni Muslim from religious persecution by the Twelver Shiite, Ismail Shah. As seen in Chapter 5, it is no mistake that these two scholars would be joined in the nineteenth century by Hamdan, an Algerian who fled French colonisation in the 1830s.[29] Each of these authors' exposure to foreign cultures may well have led to greater openness to novel conceptions of plague, preventative measures and prescriptions. Among the early Ottoman treatise writers, one can see this tendency when Al-Yahudi cited Christian doctors who prescribed untraditional, seemingly prohibited cures like alcohol, and when Bitlisi made a pitch for quicksilver, a non-Galenic chemical treatment.[30]

Strikingly, the comparative notion of judging an 'other' civilisation as the origin of an epidemic disease was also not limited to European authors. Admittedly, even the ancient Greek Thucydides, the fabled 'father of history', contended that the plague that struck Athens in 430 BCE originated in East Africa and travelled to Greece via Egypt and Persia.[31] Fourteenth-century European writers likewise believed that the Black Death came from central Asia.[32]

In contrast, Bitlisi claimed that syphilis came from Europe. Such a claim may well have stemmed from a shared dialectical tradition of 'otherness' that went back to the ancient Greeks, but the growing exposure between various global cultures must also have played a role. Syphilis indeed broke out during a time of transatlantic travel and the beginnings of European expansion. Just as the Ottomans would blame syphilis on the Europeans, so too the Europeans asserted that syphilis originated in America. This multi-layered discourse reveals that such writers conveyed their own biases, comparing one 'civilisation' with another. This comparative approach developed even further in the late eighteenth and nineteenth centuries, when reformers and/or colonist-minded European thinkers often contrasted their own 'progressive' 'modern' agenda with that of the 'backward' past. Thus, 'facts', 'witness accounts' and 'observations' about the origins of disease, or how one should react to it, have a long history of being socially constructed. Seemingly, ancient Greeks, Western orientalists and Muslim innovators have all been more than happy to construct such myths.[33]

QUARANTINES AND MERCANTILIST DISCOURSE

The development of quarantines among the maritime powers of Europe in the seventeenth and eighteenth centuries was pivotal to changes in medical treatise discourses on plague. These states adopted contagionist measures as part of a general mercantilist policy of state-led commercial and economic reforms aimed at controlling overseas trade routes by monopolising markets in which they would import raw material goods, export manufactured products and maintain a favourable balance of trade.[34] Such states, particularly Britain, Holland and France, began by developing their navies of 'ships of the line', seaworthy, ocean-going vessels with the most up-to-date cannonry, as well as their merchant marines of new, flat-bottomed sailing vessels that allowed for a far greater volume of bulk goods. These states thereafter initiated a series of reforms – establishing monopolistic trading companies, levying tariffs against foreign goods, subsidising overseas commercial commerce, promoting new credit institutions – in order to achieve their agenda.[35]

Establishing quarantines helped to justify these policies of state intervention, particularly in the Ottoman Empire, which many Europeans imagined being as plague-ridden since the 1347–8 outbreak passed through Constantinople and Cairo. It was no accident that the quarantine official who met the trading vessels on the docks, was also frequently charged with taking customs and enforcing trade monopolies. Mercantilist states often exercised sovereignty by controlling the economy in the name of public health.[36]

The plague treatise writers who debated quarantine and other preventive measures in a mercantilist context played a fundamentally different role to that which they had previously. Beforehand, plague treatise writers were tied to relatively limited court and academic circles. Some, like Fracastoro, may have entertained the idea of contagion, but they did not translate those ideas into institutions. For example, Italian city-states like Venice, Genoa and Leghorn may have regularly quarantined vessels for up to forty days from the late fourteenth to the sixteenth century, and in about 1600 may have even developed public health offices, permanent lazarettos and cadastral records of the plague dead. But there was no broad debate in print involving said state officials, plague thinkers and the merchant community. In sum, literary elites remained aloof from popular and state efforts at quarantines, even in the decades after Fracastoro's death.

Once the quarantines were established in the Atlantic mercantilist communities of north-western Europe, new commercial interests began to question the efficiency of such measures – especially if they perceived quarantine to be eating into their profits. Medical treatise writers often themselves participated in merchant ventures or were partisans of state reforms. In either case, the writers and their works aimed at this newly emerging public sphere. It was at this time that the writers first really made use of printed books, pamphlets and commercial gazettes to sell their ideas to their rapidly expanding readership.[37]

One really witnesses the beginning of such debates in London during the seventeenth and eighteenth centuries, when plague treatise writers began to participate themselves in formulating new state policies on plague, trade and overseas commercial ventures. One can see this, for instance, when members of the College of Physicians, such as Dr Richard Mead, called for quarantine measures and met responses from state officials, like Sir James Porter, long-time British Ambassador to the Porte, members of the merchant community, such as the British Levant Company's Dr Patrick Russell, and even reformist-minded critics, like John Howard.[38] London's commercial elites and booming urban economy were dependent on a powerful navy and merchant marine opening the way for overseas trade, such as with the Ottoman Empire. Their overseas trade with such places certainly played a great role in generating new wealth, particularly by providing an emerging British textile industry with bulk goods, such as cotton, wool, flax and silk. However, they also brought new public health problems to the fore. Extensive contacts with distant foreign lands were a conduit for dangerous new epidemics. Advocates of quarantines did not forget that most European accounts of the Black Death claimed that the disease came through the eastern Mediterranean and Constantinople, after it first broke out in central Asia. More recent literature on syphilis pointed to the European exploration of America as a cause for epidemics. The numerous Native American deaths the Europeans saw from smallpox were just one reminder of this trend. They also were aware that the drawbacks of London's rapid urban growth – congestion, filthy conditions, immigration and social change – often could also foster disease and death. Many saw these developments as the causes behind the plague of 1665, and the great fire that followed it in 1666.[39]

In response, English statesmen and politicians began to take new protectionist measures in order to address these concerns, thereby promoting the country's commercial and demographic development. Some of these measures, like the Bills of Mortality, which calculated London's death rate, satisfied both the statesmen and the merchants. On the one hand, the Bills were seen important for determining to what extent plague endangered the population, and led to possible preventative measures (for example, travel restrictions, quarantine and sanitary improvements). In fact, John Graunt attempted to write the first statistical survey of London based on these figures in 1661. This work and others like it would lay the groundwork for later demographic studies, better known at the time as 'political arithmetic'. On the other hand, the Bills led to greater commercial development, since they allowed people to draw up life insurance based on the death rate. This provided investors with greater financial security, and holders even began to use their policies as a form of paper currency. This helped to alleviate England's dependency on precious metal coinage, a major problem in all early modern economies. It also paved the way for even greater developments, such as stocks and bonds which fuelled London's rise as the world's pre-eminent financial capital, and the headquarters of commercial and industrial revolution.[40]

Quarantine restrictions relating to trade would prove to be far more controversial. The Royal College of Physicians recommended as early as 1636, that:

> care be taken that neither man nor goods may come from any suspected places beyond the seas, or in the land, without a certificate of health, or else either to be sent suddenly away, or to be put to the pest-house, or suchlike place, for forty days (according to the custom of Italy).[41]

In times of emergency, such as London's Great Plague of 1665, royal authority enforced such quarantines. Merchants might have protested the measure, but were reassured that it would be dropped after the plague subsided.[42]

After the plague broke out in Marseilles in 1720, the Royal College of Physicians, having now gained greater standing as a state institution, pushed for a permanently enforced quarantine. The main culprit, they maintained, were imported goods from the Ottoman Empire, including cotton and flax (from Cairo and Syria), wool (from central Anatolia) and silk (from Bursa). Not accidentally, these items made up the bulk of England's Levant trade, and were key to her textile industry.[43] Dr Mead, the chief author of the measure, saw:

> that of all the goods which harbour infection, cotton in particular is the most dangerous, and Turkey is almost a perpetual seminary of the plague; I cannot but think it highly reasonable, that whatever cotton is imported from that part of the world, should at all times be kept in quarantine; because it may have imbibed infection at the time of its packing up, not withstanding no mischief has been felt from it by the ship's company.[44]

England's commercial elites, particularly Levant Company partisans, bitterly protested this restriction, arguing that the merchants and sailors involved in the trade would surely have been the plague's first victims if cotton, and other like porous items, were indeed infectious:

> The merchants who have lived in Turkey can inform us, that after the plague has ceased, they, or their servants, do handle and smell the cotton etc. without receiving any injury. Every one who has been in Turkey well knows that stevedores and sailors often work naked, in stowing the cotton. This is a laborious employment, and the hold of the ship is excessive hot. Further, the cotton packs or bales are continually handled and tumbled about; the labourers too are often bare footed, therefore they cannot help treading continually on the merchandise brought aboard.[45]

Others asserted that the plague was never transmitted in England from the Ottoman Empire, as it was endemic to that country alone:

> Has not merchandise been brought from many parts of Turkey, all which have very deservedly an ill name for the pestilence, that very commonly rages among them? And how comes it to pass that during this constant, and uninterrupted commerce, when soft and porous goods, the proper somes, have been brought from Smyrna, Iskenderun, Aleppo, Constantinople, and other parts, the pestilence has never taken a journey hither, in all appearance, those fifty-five years [since the Great Plague of 1665]?[46]

There were even some who claimed that the quarantine of goods could spell the end of England as a mercantile power:

> The Venetians (says a certain author) were long possessed of the profitable Turkey trade, and were almost the only merchants that traded into Turkey,

> and furnished the western parts of Europe with this merchandise; in all that time they had no notions of the frequent plagues being conveyed in goods they brought home, and were transported into other nations. And it is very remarkable, that about the time they instituted officers of health, and begun the practice of quarantines . . . their trade fell sensibly into decay. Our merchants about the same time made experiments of the Turkey trade, and became proselytes to this Turkish opinion, that a plague is not conveyed in goods.[47]

This passage illustrates the fear that quarantines established in England would be a devastating public expense and bureaucratisation that would kill trade and play into the hands of the country's commercial rivals.

Parliament ignored most of these protests when it passed Mead's Quarantine Act in 1721. Although they did not establish lazarettos in England proper, British government officials, acting through their Ottoman consulate, would judge whether a quarantine of varying lengths needed to be carried out at a number of Mediterranean ports (for example, Malta, Ancona, Messina, Venice, Leghorn and Marseilles). If there were no rumoured or confirmed cases of plague, the British officials could issue a 'clean bill of health' meaning that the ship would either be exempt from quarantine or only required to wait up to two weeks in one of the lazarettos. However, if there were concerns about plague, the British Consul would issue a 'foul bill of health', requiring a full quarantine of forty days.[48]

New protests soon circulated against these measures. Some, like James Porter, a former British Ambassador resident in Istanbul, stated categorically that he had never heard of plague affecting any of his countrymen:

> There is not, indeed, upon record, nor has a single living witness ever related an instance of an English factor, or servant's dying of the plague at any of the seaport towns, or in any other part of Syria, or Asia Minor, but only one at Constantinople, in almost a century; though the disease frequently rages in that metropolis.[49]

Such statements may have led to arguments about the innate superior health of the British, or perhaps the benefits of the British diet or hygiene. The main point, however, was that the British should waste no time bothering about contagionist measures, as it would only hurt the Levant Company's profits.

Others claimed that the methods used for quarantining merchandise, such as the airing of cotton, actually damaged the product. John Howard, the late eighteenth-century reformist who generally advocated for stricter quarantine measures, admitted this himself:

> The cottons are taken out of the bags containing them, and placed in rows of piles, upon boards lay down on stone pillars about 18 inches from the floors; and in repacking they are flung over a man who gets into the bags, in order to tread down the cotton; the consequence of which must be exposing him to greater danger should any infection remain. This, though the surest way of expelling infection from cotton, is not the most agreeable to merchants, not only because more expensive, but also [because it damages the merchandise].[50]

Yet another popular argument among the merchants was that the Levant Company and the local consul needed no further governmental supervision after loading in port. Porter argued, for instance, that the merchants took extremely vigilant measures to protect themselves from the epidemic disease:

> All communication of the infection must arise either from men or merchandise; with regard to the former, when there is the least suspicion of plague in any seaport town of Turkey or any neighbouring village, the master of ships, the merchants, and the consul are particularly careful and vigilant to keep the vessel at a proper distance in the port, and not to suffer any of the ship's company to go on shore; at the same time they will not permit a living soul to come aboard, or any good susceptible to infection to approach the vessel. All seamen are strictly forbidden to go near it; and, to do them justice, they punctually obey the order: for when the fear of that disease is once infused into their minds, they dread it more than a wreck, or a cannon ball.[51]

Porter's logic here was that a merchant ship's crew were well aware that the journey from the Ottoman Empire to England would take at least two months. Plague would rapidly spread in the stagnant air of the ship's cabin, typically killing from a half to two-thirds of the crew before arrival.[52]

Also popular, of course, were appeals to British patriotism. Porter lauded his own countrymen's survival instincts as a supreme virtue:

> The desire of self-preservation is as strongly implanted in the breast of an Englishman; it actuates him as powerfully abroad as at home; he would not surely venture the loss of his life by infection, if there were the least grounds for such apprehension.[53]

Such statements would seem powerful, especially given the sentiments of many Members of Parliament who would decide on the matter, since they too were sympathetic to commercial interests, often holding stocks or participating in the trade directly.[54]

John Russell, himself a factor of the Levant Company, and, interestingly, a doctor of medicine who supported Mead's Quarantine Act, stopped short of accusing his fellow merchants of reckless greed:

> He must entertain an ill opinion of mankind who can believe any merchant, in the Levant, from lucrative motives, would risk the health of his country, by exporting merchandise when the plague was raging in the place; or under the conviction of his own mind, that his commerce, highly advantageous as it might be to himself, might in the event involve thousands of his fellow creatures in misery.[55]

Patriotic appeals reached their height when it came to trade rivalries, however. The English merchants almost invariably compared their own trade with that of the Dutch, whose merchant marine and commercial economy competed with the English throughout the seventeenth and early eighteenth centuries. The Dutch were the undoubted pioneers of free trade and were even more reluctant than the British to adopt quarantines. James Porter jealously argued that:

> The Dutch never receive the contagion directly from thence [the Ottoman Empire]; they have admitted ships into their ports, either with clean or foul bills of health, and found themselves, as we may, always safe.[56]

Howard took an entirely different tack when he blamed the great plague of 1665 on these free-wheeling Dutch traders:

> I do not hesitate to affirm, from the fullest authority of undeniable testimony, that it first entered this island by means of contagion, and was brought from Holland in merchandise imported from that country, where it had made great ravages the preceding year; and if anyone is desirous of inquiring further into its origin, I inform him, that if any credit is to be given to report, its seeds were brought into Holland from the Turkish empire, along with cotton, which is a most faithful preserver of contagion.[57]

Howard's argument was highly provocative, given the growing importance of Levant cotton in the late eighteenth century. When Mead first pushed for his Quarantine Act in 1720, cotton was not nearly as important to the Levant Company, as their import trade favoured silk, followed by other raw material commodities like cotton. The British cotton textile industry was only just developing at that time, and its demand was largely met by American and Caribbean cotton producers. When Howard wrote in 1787, the situation had dramatically changed. The newly independent United States, along with their French and

Spanish supporters, did not guarantee the British unfettered access to their colonial supplies of cotton at a time when demand was soaring. Rapid technological improvements in the 1770s and 1780s transformed England's cotton textile production into one of the main engines of the Industrial Revolution.[58]

Howard furthermore claimed that the Dutch refused to build their own lazaretto to protect the public:

> When representations were made in Holland on the necessity of establishing a lazaretto to obviate this risk, and the fatal consequences which the introduction of the plague might be to all of Europe; but perhaps the Hollanders, ever preferring the interests of their trade to those of humanity, would not allow so forcible an argument to have any weight with them; but gave for answer, that it would be time enough to think of a lazaretto when English had built one.[59]

This picture took on an even more sinister tone when one considers the Dutch outsourced up to three-quarters of their cotton trade to the Ottoman Greek minority, who were granted the right to fly the Dutch flag on their trading vessels.[60] The Greeks, who made up a substantial community in almost all the major Ottoman ports, would often give:

> False reports concerning the plague . . . Their deputies inform consuls of accidents having happened in their nation, when in reality there is no plague in this city or its environs.[61]

Such criminal activity would depress their British rivals since they would have to:

> Perform a long and expensive quarantine in the ports of the Mediterranean, by which means the cottons which form their principal loading, as well as the chief article of both trades, are no less than seven months on their way to London.[62]

In contrast, the Greeks could quickly move their ships to Holland, where they would perform a minimal quarantine, if at all. All told, the Greek ships could deliver their cargo at least two to three months before their British rivals. This allowed the Dutch to supply more than half of the Ottoman cotton to London. Thus, the British quarantine would be compromised by lax Dutch measures and potentially contaminated cotton.[63] At least some of the supporters of the 1721 legislation, such as Daniel Defoe, had this loophole in mind, as it supported the Channel and Atlantic cotton trades at the expense of the Levant Company.[64] By the 1780s, this favouritism was no longer in the national interest, since the War of American Independence had cut England off from French, American and Caribbean supplies.[65]

John Howard's answer to this conundrum was to establish a permanent lazaretto in England, which all arriving ships would have to undergo. He also called for a ban on third-party cotton trade, which in effect meant a shipping monopoly for the Levant Company, since the Navigation Acts strictly prohibited foreign vessels from trading in English ports. Howard sought the measures in order to secure the country's public health by limiting the risk to plague; but he also argued that they would have a profoundly positive effect in promoting British trade:

> In what a different situation would the establishment of a lazaretto put it? By depriving the Dutch of the advantages they now enjoy, we should be able to supply the whole quantity of cottons demanded at our market; instead of only sending 5,000 bales, we should send more than double that quantity annually; and as by a fixed regulation of the Levant Company, we can only purchase the products of this country with the produce of goods sent from England, the importation of our manufactures would increase in the same proportion. The quantity of shipping employed in the trade would likewise be doubled, and by earning the freight which is now paid to the Dutch, on the cottons they sent to England, it would be so much clearer gain to the nation, added to the advantages which would attend the extension of its navigation, an increase of the consumption of its manufacturers; advantages which are now enjoyed by our rivals the Dutch, the prosperity of whose trade is founded on the ruin of ours.[66]

The argument that a mandatory national lazaretto would double British cotton shipments and increase exports assumed British textile factories would continue to flood the market even after implementing the quarantine. Regardless of the uniformity the measures might create in terms of regulating the trade, the lag time of up to seven months per shipment would not change.[67] Nevertheless, the British did not have to worry about foreign competition, since their navy ruled the Mediterranean after Admiral Horatio Nelson's defeat of Napoleon's fleet at the Battle of the Nile in 1798. Likewise, the national interest would not be harmed if British textile factory owners abandoned the Ottoman cotton market for India, where the British East India Company largely dominated cotton production.[68]

In general, mercantilist plague treatise writers – both quarantine advocates and opponents – were much more connected to the public sphere, particularly with regard to commercial and trading interests. In 1665, Dr Hodges speculated that Dutch imported cotton caused London's Great Plague, an easy enough argument when the English were in the midst of a war with the Netherlands.[69] In

1720, Daniel Defoe would condemn the Levant Company and Dr Mead would claim that the Ottoman Empire was the seminary of the plague; both played key roles in shaping quarantine legislation that favoured non-Levant trading interests. Similarly, mandatory lazarettos were established by 1788 in part to secure new sources of cotton and further nationalise trade.[70] Yet, from the 1670s onwards, there was not a single plague death recorded in London's Bills of Mortality.[71] It would seem that profit rates, not death rates, were the bottom line to quarantine reform discussions.

AN OTTOMAN RESPONSE?

The issue to consider, then, is why the Ottomans did not adopt a quarantine until the 1830s. One might expect the Ottomans to have developed initial measures as early as the sixteenth century, given the concentration of plague writers, undoubted social and administrative innovations, and their proximity and interaction with Venice, Ragusa and other Italian city-states that had started quarantines of their own. At least one European observer, Ogier Ghiselin de Busbecq, the Holy Roman Empire's ambassador to Istanbul between 1554 and 1562 believed that the Ottomans dogmatic resistance to innovation explained this discrepancy:

> The populace at large rejected the idea of contagion on the grounds 'that the time and manner of each man's death is inscribed by God upon his forehead; if, therefore, he is destined to die, it is useless for him to try to avert fate; if he is not so destined, he is foolish to be afraid'.[72]

There is also no evidence of quarantine reform among the vast numbers of cadastral records governing land, revenue and administrative control during the mid-sixteenth century, even though key Ottoman Muslim authorities like Ebussuud were amenable to flight and other medical precautions to avoid plague.[73]

Yet geopolitical factors, such as the Ottoman loss of sea power, also need to be considered. Quarantine reform in Europe was developed in order to protect and promote overseas commercial trade, but had no relevance to the Ottomans after they had largely ceded control over much of the Mediterranean, Red Sea and Indian Ocean and made no efforts to match the European expansion into the Atlantic and Pacific. The Ottomans, in contrast to European powers like the English, could not use a substantial merchant marine to modernise its economy and create new commercial links which increased wealth and, incidentally, biological links with the outside world.[74]

Overseas European merchant communities in the major Ottoman ports of Istanbul, Izmir, Beirut and Cairo began to impose their own quarantine. For example, Alexander Russell, a British trader to the Ottoman trading hub of Aleppo wrote in 1744 that:

> Next to the protection of Divine Providence, the means that the Europeans depend upon for their preservation during the time of plague [in Aleppo], consist either in a retreat from the city, or in setting up in their town houses, in such a manner as effectively to prevent all intercourse or communication by which the infection might be received from without.[75]

In Russell's opinion:

> The advantages of shutting up, are in that country fully confirmed by experience, so that all the Christians and Jews . . . followed the example of the Franks; and even . . . the Turks (who on account of an avowed principle of religion, cannot openly adopt the custom). Many of those particularly conversant with Europeans, devise various pretexts for keeping much at home; sometimes they retire to one of their garden houses, as if merely on a party of pleasure; at other times, when their affairs will permit, they make a commercial excursion to some distant city: A journey to Mecca, under the pretence of devotion, is no unusual expedient for avoiding the impending danger.[76]

Such statements led people to believe that it was only the Europeans or 'Franks' who could really regulate health and, by insinuation, good government.

In actuality, the Ottomans actually went further with plague control measures than most scholars give credit for. While they did not have Bills of Mortality or cadastral Books of the Dead as found in seventeenth-century England and Florence, one can see certain tendencies that led in this direction. For instance, Molla Mustafa Ševki Bašeski, a local Ottoman Muslim notable from Sarajevo, chronicles numerous instances of the plague which hit his city in 1746 and the following years. In his book he records the name, number and the profession of each of the victims. Although his work was not a formal record of the city's dead, I would maintain that one might find similar records in other Ottoman urban centres of that era.[77]

As we can see from Dr Richard Mead, the author of the 1721 British Quarantine Act, the Ottoman treatise writers were probably not the only ones to believe in contagion:

> The late Mr. Williams, chaplain to Sir Robert Sutton, when Ambassador at Constantinople [from 1710 to 1714] used to relate a story of the same nature told him by a pasha: that in an expedition this pasha made to the frontiers of Poland,

> one of the janissaries under his command died of the plague; whose jacket, a very rich one, had been bought by another janissary, it was no sooner put on, but he also was taken sick and died: and this same misfortune befell five janissaries more who afterwards wore it. This the pasha related to Mr. Williams, chiefly for the sake of this further circumstance, that the incidents now mentioned prevailed upon him to order the burning of the garment: designing by this instance to let Mr. Williams see there were Turks who allowed themselves in so much freedom of thought, as not to pay that strict regard to the Mohammedan doctrine of fatalism, as the vulgar among them do.[78]

Ironically, Mead cites a Turk as an example to his British audience, especially given his belief that the Ottoman Empire was 'the seminary of the plague'.[79] Moreover, the fact that the pasha supposedly related the tale to Mr Williams indicates the possibility that key Ottoman notables and statesman might have implemented quarantine reform if given the chance.

An anonymous British writer soon shot back a counter-argument:

> Where should be the wonder, to see several people dying in the same coat, in times of pestilence. It is really no more than if several men became heirs to the same estate, one after another successively, as the Turks reason. The true state of this question is, whether the men had the plague before they put on the coat? Or that they died by putting it on? The last is impossible; because of the suddenness of the death, and supposing them otherwise in good health: and the former is the case common enough in times of pestilence, as we may learn by making a voyage to Turkey; where we may find coats of all sorts, belonging to many masters, without describing the cause of their death to the habit.[80]

Here the author posited that most Turks realised the non-contagious nature of plague. Like Mead, he also cited the Turks in high regard, in contradistinction to many negative comparisons, particularly in the late eighteenth and nineteenth centuries. He also indicated the increasing contagionist/anti-contagionist debate, and that Turkish anti-contagionists should not be simply seen as vulgar fatalists as Dr Mead asserted.

One instance where the anti-contagionist belief in the environmental, miasmatic nature of plague led to new innovations was in sanitary reforms. For instance, Ahmed Efendi, an Ottoman astrologer, related the following story about the plague and Istanbul's city planning in 1708:

> One day after an earthquake the Sultan gathered philosophers together and asked them how they could stop it. The learned men said that they could solve the

> problem but that the solution would cause plague. By building underground reservoirs (*sertablar*) you could prevent earthquakes since the fumes would gather there. Wells are also vulnerable to this. The reservoirs, however, would generate fetid air, which would result in plague. The Sultan responded that it was better to have this solution since outbreaks of plague were better than earthquakes. You could cure plague with medicine but an earthquake would kill up to a hundred thousand and damage the buildings. Now days few of these underground reservoirs are left.[81]

This story is evidence that earthquakes and fires were seen by the Ottoman sultan and the authorities as a greater danger to the city than plague. Nevertheless, the later improvements that were made, such as fresh running water, were seen as preventing plague. This is not dissimilar to sanitary movements that you would see elsewhere, such as in London after the Great Fire of 1666.[82]

One outside admirer of Ottoman sanitation was James DeKay, a gifted American traveller who resided in Istanbul in 1831 and 1832 and who acquired an extensive knowledge of the language, culture and society of the people there. DeKay was greatly impressed by the Ottoman capital's water works in comparison with cities in the United States:

> Every stranger is struck with numerous contrivances around Constantinople for supplying it with pure and wholesome water. Belonging to a city in the United States which has long been distinguished for its nauseous and detestable water, and for the culpable negligence of its rulers on a subject of so much importance, no opportunity was neglected to obtain all the information in our power in regard to the hydraulic establishments in this neighborhood. The result, however mortifying, must not be concealed, and we therefore state, that on a subject intimately connected, not only with the comfort, but with the health of the people, the commercial emporium of the United States is some centuries behind the metropolis of Turkey.[83]

He later concluded that Istanbul's waterworks must be at least 50 miles long and worth more than $50 million (in 1831). In contrast he also asserted that:

> The City of New York, with a population of more than 200,000 inhabitants, has been deliberating for years over the question – whether it is expedient to spend two millions of dollars for the purpose of introducing a copious supply of pure and wholesome water.[84]

DeKay made several important observations about the commitment of the Ottoman government to public health. First he claimed that the Ottoman state maintained a strong and continuous effort to maintain the water works. A separate governmental supervisor, and even the head of state often exercised direct control:

> So important are these watercourses considered that the sultans have always been in the habit of making annually a formal visit of inspection, which is accompanied with much ceremony, and ordering such improvements and alterations as are deemed necessary.[85]

DeKay extensively described a water reservoir. He indicated that there were many such constructions in the mid- to late eighteenth century, which again substantiates Ahmed Efendi's earlier story. One should also note, however, that the water works were also substantially developed from 1550 to 1560, when the population of Istanbul grew from 150,000 to 600,000. There is extensive documentary evidence that a water inspectorate was founded to regulate the water works. Still, the Ottoman bureaucracy often had to maintain a careful balance between their desire for regularising control over the capital and the popular push for greater rights and privileges over this precious resource.[86] This political tension was contrary to DeKay's contention that the sultan exercised absolute control of the water.

Nevertheless, there is much to be said for DeKay's observations on innovating the waterways. He, unlike many Western visitors, credited the Ottomans with improving the city. In contrast to the Roman and Byzantine aqueducts and reservoirs, which at the time he wrote had long 'gone into disuse, as expensive and inadequate for the purposes intended',[87] the Ottomans had invented a system of pipes and pillars that collected running water more efficiently from the hillsides around Istanbul:

> They form a striking peculiarity in Turkish scenery, and it was some time before the principle upon which they were constructed was apparent. The water leaves the brow of a hill, and descending in earth and pipes rises in leaden or earthen ones, up one side of this pillar, to its former level, which must be, of course, the summit of the pillar, or *sooteray*, as it is called by the Turks. The water is here discharged into a stone basin as large as the top of the *sooteray*, and is discharged by another pipe, which descends along the opposite side of the pillar, enters the ground, advances to the next *sooteray*, which it ascends and descends in the same manner; in this way the level of the water may be preserved for many miles over a large plain, when an aqueduct would be, from its expansiveness, manifestly out of the question. In the city of Constantinople, the old aqueducts that no longer conduct water in the usual manner, are converted into a series of *sooterays*, and permits one to examine their structure in detail.[88]

DeKay then proceeds to describe the unique features of the invention, with an eye on possibly adopting it back home in the United States:

> This ingenious hydraulic arrangement seems to possess advantages which might recommend its adoption elsewhere. As the pressure is thus divided among this series of siphons, the necessity for having very strong and costly pipes is obviated. As they are from 300 to 500 yards apart, the cost is probably much less than by any plan which could be devised, where, in addition to the cost of a canal or a series of pipes, we should be compelled to raise it again by the expensive agency of steam or some other costly apparatus. The frequent exposure of the water to air and light at the summit of these *sooterays* is another important advantage which cannot be too strongly insisted upon; as it is now well known that nothing tends more to purify water than the presence of these two agents. The arrangement likewise of the basins on the top of the pillars is well adapted for getting rid of much of the matters deposited from turbid waters. Lastly to the descending pipe a small cock is attached near the ground, by which the flocks and herds of the adjoining villages and fields are furnished at all times with a copious supply of water.[89]

While many might look at the DeKay's argument as a fanciful, one should not forget that traveller's accounts often led to a new innovative designs, such as the British adoption of smallpox inoculations after Lady Montagu's description in 1718 of how Turkish village women injected infected tissue into their veins in order to prevent the disease.[90] Whether DeKay's *sooteray* was actually adopted in New York after his visit to Istanbul deserves further investigation.

DeKay did not end his account without highlighting the Ottoman state's commitment to the welfare of its people. This was most evident when he saw that no one ruler ever claimed much credit for the water works:

> They [the fountains] are frequently decorated with the inscription setting forth the greatness and goodness of Providence, and inviting the weary traveller to make due acknowledgements for the same. Unlike our civilized ostentation, the name of the benevolent constructor never appears on these sculptured stones. The quaint Turkish adage, which serves as a rule of conduct, is well exemplified in this as well as in many other instances: 'Do good and throw it into the sea; if the fishes don't know it, God will'.[91]

This goes to one of his main arguments: namely, that although the Ottomans' belief in the general welfare of their people may have had its basis in the Islamic faith, it was also reflective of enlightened Western values.

As DeKay's account shows, the Ottomans of the seventeenth and eighteenth centuries were not focused on undertaking quarantine reform. Works by Ottoman plague treatise writers during this time – like those written by Bašeski or Ahmed Efendi – were few and far between. Ottoman statesmen and administrators may have supported public health works, such as Istanbul's water supplies, but this was a sanitary, anti-contagionist measure unconnected with the treatise writers or commercial elites. This trend would change only when the mercantilist European powers who did adopt quarantines began to challenge the Empire's sovereignty in the name of public health.

CONCLUSION

Indeed, before the development of the mercantile colonialist states European and Middle Eastern Muslim plague treatise writers strongly resembled each other. Muslim writers, from the fourteenth-century Andalusians Al-Khatimah and Al-Khatib to fifteenth- and sixteenth-century Ottoman writers like Al-Yahudi, Bitlisi and Taşköprüzade, were just as receptive to innovation and contagionist thought as their European counterparts, Fracastoro included. That Fracastoro had his work printed rather than relying solely on penned copies does not belie the fact that these Ottoman and European authors still appealed to relatively limited audiences.[92]

Mercantile development, particularly in England, fundamentally changed the equation by commercialising the plague treatise writer and his product. The English plague treatise writer, for example, produced his work with the emerging market of economic ideas in mind. The conflict of contagionist and anti-contagionist thought continued to bear a superficial resemblance to earlier debates, but the process of social construction was far more subtle. The writer's work was ever more aimed at overseas commercial interests. Remembering Adam Smith, one might postulate that these writers, like the everyday British labourer or business professional, was going through a process of specialisation that would lead to a career as a public health official, state reformer or commercial lobbyist.[93] Their arguments would either suit the utilitarianism interests of these concerns or risk being discarded. Whether Parliament or the Crown accepted or patronised quarantine proposals, such as Dr Mead's Quarantine Act of 1721 or John Howard's late eighteenth-century proposed mandatory lazaretto, depended upon the market realities of that time. Ideas could change because of many economic factors, such as company monopolies, war, and a growing need for cotton and other 'dangerous' raw material goods.

The Ottoman plague treatise writers between 1600 and 1800 pale in comparison. Not only were there very few new works composed during this time, but there also was no comparable drive for mercantilist reform. Ottoman statesmen, like the pasha mentioned in Dr Mead's account or Bašeski, might have entertained ideas of contagionist reform, but they lacked commercial interest and the support of the Ottoman state.[94] The government undoubtedly made great strides towards improved public health and kept an open mind with regard to innovation, as can seen in the *sooterays* and the other water-works reforms. Still, the only quarantines in the Ottoman Empire were run by European expatriates and the Greek minority, which apparently also saw the economic utility of the institution. Quarantine also served a useful ideological function for these groups as well: namely, as a marker to distinguish themselves from the fatalistic, barbarian, Ottoman 'other'. Such orientalist discourse would prove to be formidable at the time of European expansion during the early nineteenth century.[95] It was only when this threat was imminent – as seen in the French invasion of Egypt and Algeria, the British support for an independent Greek state, and the unequal commercial treaty of Balta Liman – that the Ottomans would respond.

NOTES

1. Giovanni Boccaccio, trans. Guido Waldman, *The Decameron*, pp. 6–14; Girolamo Fracastoro, *De Contagione et Contagiosis Morbis et Eorum Curatione, Libri III*, p. 3.
2. Panzac, *La Peste dans l'Empire Ottoman*, pp. 312–39.
3. Dols, *The Black Death in the Middle East*, pp. 9–12; David Herlihy, *Black Death and the Transformation of the West*, pp. 40–1.
4. Boccaccio, *The Decameron*, p. 2.
5. Boccaccio, *The Decameron*, p. 3.
6. Herlihy, pp. 71–2.
7. Vivian Nutton, 'The Reception of Fracastoro's Theory of Contagion: The Seed that Fell Among Thorns?', pp. 203–5, 210, 214–16.
8. Anna Campbell, *The Black Death and Men of Learning*, pp. 50–6, 69–72, 79–86.
9. Campbell, *The Black Death and Men of Learning*, pp. 66–73, 86–8.
10. Campbell, *The Black Death and Men of Learning*, p. 57.
11. Dols, *The Black Death in the Middle East*, pp. 92–4; Ulmann, *Islamic Medicine*, p. 94.
12. Ulmann, *Islamic Medicine*, p. 94.
13. Roy Porter, *The Greatest Benefit to Mankind: A Medical History of Humanity from Antiquity to the Present*, pp. 238–41, 428–9.
14. Vivian Nutton, 'Seeds of Disease: An Explanation of Contagion and Infection from the Greeks to the Renaissance', pp. 1–2, 33–4.
15. Dols, *The Black Death in the Middle East*, pp. 92–4; Ulmann, *Islamic Medicine*, p. 93.
16. Bitlisi, *Hısn ül-veba*, fol. 29A.
17. Al-Yahudi, *Micennetü't-Ta'un ve'l-Veba*, fols 11A, 13B–20A; Bitlisi, *Hısn ül-veba*, fol. 27A; Müstakimzade, *Cihazü'l-Macun fi'l-Halas Mine't-Taun*, fols 48A–B; Osman, *Tercüme-i İthaf*, fol. 15A.
18. See Chapter 2, pp. 15–19, 24–8.

19. Müstakimzade, *Cihazü'l-Macun fi'l-Halas Mine't-Taun*, fol. 47B; Al-Yahudi, *Micennetü't-Ta'un ve'l-Veba*, fols 9A–13A, 15A.
20. Derviş Abdullah, *Müfredat*, fol. 104A.
21. Bitlisi, *Hısn ül-veba*, fols 27B–28A.
22. Bernard Lewis, *What Went Wrong? Western Impact and Middle Eastern Response*, pp. 39, 80–1; Bernard Lewis, *The Muslim Discovery of Europe*, pp. 227–31.
23. Berkes, *The Development of Secularism in Turkey*, p. 113.
24. Al-Yahudi, *Micennetü't-Ta'un ve'l-Veba*, fols 1A–B; Bitlisi, *Hısn ül-veba*, fols 2A–6B.
25. Vivian Nutton, 'Books, Printing and Medicine in the Renaissance', pp. 434–5; Roy Porter, *Greatest Benefit to Mankind*, pp. 72–4; Sam White, *The Climate of Rebellion in the Early Modern Ottoman Empire*, pp. 85–7.
26. Ebussuud; Abdulgani.
27. Nutton, 'Books', pp. 422, 432.
28. Edmond Gibbon, *The Decline and Fall of the Roman Empire*, abridged by D. M. Low, pp. 712–18. Even today, authors like Bernard Lewis make the claim that Sephardic Jewish doctors who fled Spain for the Ottoman Empire, such as Al-Yahudi, brought valuable know-how to a scientifically starved empire. In his eyes, their effect was limited, as they were gradually assimilated into Islamic, tradition-bound ways. Lewis, *Muslim Discovery*, p. 230.
29. See Chapter 5, pp. 100–12.
30. Al-Yahudi, *Micennetü't-Ta'un ve'l-Veba*, fols 9A–13A; Bitlisi, *Hısn ül-veba*, fols 27B–8A.
31. Thucydides, *The History of the Peloponnesian War, by Thucydides. A New and Literal Version, from the Text of Arnold, Collated with Bekker, Göller, and Poppo*, pp. 30–4.
32. Samuel K. Cohn Jr. *The Black Death Transformed: Disease and Culture in early Renaissance Europe*, p. 102.
33. Gibbon, *Decline and Fall of the Roman Empire*, pp. 712–18, 820–32; Lewis, *Muslim Discovery*, pp. 228–9; Dols, *The Black Death in the Middle East*, pp. 92–4, 110–20.
34. William Coleman, *Yellow Fever in the North*, pp. 87–90.
35. Paul Langford, *A Polite and Commercial People: England, 1727–1783*, pp. 2–7.
36. Panzac, *La Peste dans l'Empire Ottoman*, pp. 117–8, 129–30; Roy Porter, *Greatest Benefit to Mankind*, pp. 236–8.
37. Nutton, 'Books', pp. 434–5; Nutton, 'Reception', pp. 232–4; Roy Porter, *The Creation of the Modern World: The Untold Story of the British Enlightenment*, pp. 72–4.
38. Howard, *Account of the Principal Lazarettos in Europe*; Mead, *A Short Discourse*; Mead, *Discourse on the Plague*; James Porter, *Observations on the Religion, Law, Government and Manners*; Patrick Russell, *A Treatise of the Plague*.
39. Campbell, *The Black Death and Men of Learning*, p. 1; Ralph Davis, *Aleppo and Devonshire Square*, pp. 13–14; Charles Henry Hull (ed.), *The Economic Writings of Sir William Petty: Together with the Observations upon the Bills of Mortality more probably by John Graunt*, pp. lxxx–lxxxii.
40. John Graunt, *Natural and Political Observations Mentioned in a Following Index, and Made upon the Bills of Mortality . . . by Capt. John Graunt*; Nathaniel Hodges, *Loimologia: or, an Historical Account of the Plague in London in 1665: With Precautionary Directions against the Like Contagion. By Nath. Hodges, M.D. . . . To which is Added, An Essay on the Different Causes of Pestilential Disease*; Hull, *The Economic Writings of Sir William Petty*, pp. lxxx–lxxxvi.

41. Patrick Russell, *A Treatise of the Plague*, p. 318, fn. 10.
42. Charles F. Mullett, 'The English Plague Scare of 1720–1721', pp. 484–516.
43. Davis, *Aleppo and Devonshire Square*, pp. 14–17.
44. Mead, *A Short Discourse*, p. 13.
45. John Kells Ingram, *A History of Political Economy*, pp. 94, 99, 72. Patrick Russell, *A Treatise of the Plague*, p. 315.
46. Explainer, *Distinct Notions of the Plague, with the Rise and Fall of Pestilential Contagion. By the Explainer*, p. 105; Patrick Russell, *A Treatise of the Plague*, p. 321.
47. Explainer, *Distinct Notions of the Plague*, p. 104; Patrick Russell, *A Treatise of the Plague* pp. 329–30.
48. Howard, *Account of the Principal Lazarettos in Europe*, p. 28; James Porter, *Observations on the Religion, Law, Government and Manners*, p. 441; Patrick Russell, *A Treatise of the Plague*, p. 343.
49. James Porter, *Observations on the Religion, Law, Government and Manners*, p. 450.
50. Howard, *Account of the Principal Lazarettos in Europe*, p. 9.
51. James Porter, *Observations on the Religion, Law, Government and Manners*, p. 442.
52. Patrick Russell, *A Treatise of the Plague* p. 349.
53. James Porter, *Observations on the Religion, Law, Government and Manners*, p. 449.
54. Davis, *Aleppo and Devonshire Square*, pp. 19–21.
55. Patrick Russell, *A Treatise of the Plague*, p. 368.
56. James Porter, *Observations on the Religion, Law, Government and Manners*, p. 441.
57. Howard, *Account of the Principal Lazarettos in Europe*, p. 32.
58. Hodges, *Loimologia*, p. 30; Charles Maclean, *Results of an Investigation Respecting Epidemic and Pestilential Diseases; Including Researches in the Levant Concerning the Plague*, pp. 1–7.
59. Howard, *Account of the Principal Lazarettos in Europe*, p. 28.
60. Howard, *Account of the Principal Lazarettos in Europe*, pp. 22, 27; Patrick Russell, *A Treatise of the Plague* p. 361.
61. Howard, *Account of the Principal Lazarettos in Europe*, p. 27.
62. Howard, *Account of the Principal Lazarettos in Europe*, p. 27.
63. Howard, *Account of the Principal Lazarettos in Europe*, p. 27.
64. Daniel Defoe, *The History of the Great Plague in London, in the Year 1665 . . . By a Citizen, Who Lived the Whole Time in London. To which is Added, a Journal of the Plague at Marseilles, in the Year 1720.*
65. Charles F. Mullett, 'Politics, Economics and Medicine: Charles Maclean and Anti-contagionism', pp. 224–51.
66. Howard, *Account of the Principal Lazarettos in Europe*, pp. 28–9.
67. Howard, *Account of the Principal Lazarettos in Europe*, p. 27.
68. Mullett, 'Politics, Economics', pp. 226, 233, 236–7, 240–3; Panzac, *La Peste dans l'Empire Ottoman*, 134–45; Howard, *Account of the Principal Lazarettos in Europe*, pp. 3–5.
69. Hodges, *Loimologia*, p. 30.
70. Daniel Defoe, *The Case Fairly Stated between the Turkey Company and the Italian Merchants*; Mead, *A Short Discourse*, p. 13.
71. Mullett, 'English Plague', pp. 485–6.
72. Lowry, 'Pushing the Stone Uphill?', p. 131.
73. Niccolo Machiavelli, *The Prince*, pp. 129–35. The conclusion most current day prominent

scholars of Ottoman science and medicine have reached is that something had dramatically 'gone wrong'. For instance, Heath Lowry's recent article on the Ottoman's reaction to plague even goes so far as to claim that 1517, some three years after Machiavelli's publication of *The Prince*, was the major turning point in Ottoman history. He claims that Sultan Yavuz Selim's victory over the Mamelukes at the Battle of Çaldıran that year and the consequent incorporation of the key Arabic lands (the Arabian peninsula, Egypt, Syria and parts of Iraq) led to the transformation of the Ottomans from pragmatic rule with a 'loose version of heterodox Islam' to dogmatic Sunni Muslims, 'the recognized leaders of the premier Orthodox Islamic state in the world'. Qualitatively, Lowry would argue that a popularly open-minded attitude towards plague as contagion and flight as an accepted preventative measure would be rejected in the decades to come. Fatalistic inaction would become the rule. Dols, *The Black Death in the Middle East*, pp. 281–302; Lewis, *Muslim Discovery*, pp. 128–30; Lowry, 'Pushing the Stone Uphill?, p. 130; Dols, *The Black Death in the Middle East*, pp. 281–302.

74. Halil İnalcık with Donald Quataert, *An Economic and Social History of the Ottoman Empire*, pp. 123, 144–6.
75. Alexander Russell, *Natural History of Aleppo, 1742–1744*, vol. 2, p. 373; Panzac, *La Peste dans l'Empire Ottoman*, p. 312.
76. Alexander Russell, *Natural History of Aleppo*, p. 376; Panzac, *La Peste dans l'Empire Ottoman*, pp. 333–4.
77. Molla Mustafa Ševki Bašeski, *Ljetopis 1749–1804*, pp. 6–7, 10, 285–7. I am grateful to Dr York Norman for pointing out this source and translating relevant passages from Bosnian to English.
78. Mead, *A Short Discourse*, p. 84.
79. Mead, *A Short Discourse*, p. 13.
80. Explainer, *Distinct Notions of the Plague*, pp. 111–12.
81. Pertev Paşa, *Risale fi İlmi Tılsım*, fols 95A–B.
82. Roy Porter, *Greatest Benefit*, p. 120.
83. James Ellsworth DeKay, *Sketches of Turkey in 1831 and 1832*, p. 110.
84. DeKay, *Sketches of Turkey*, p. 117.
85. DeKay, *Sketches of Turkey*, p. 111.
86. Robert Mantran, *17. Yüzyılın İkinci Yarısında İstanbul*, vol. 1, pp. 45–48.
87. DeKay, *Sketches of Turkey*, pp. 110–11.
88. DeKay, *Sketches of Turkey*, pp. 115–16.
89. DeKay, *Sketches of Turkey*, pp. 116–17.
90. Lady Mary Wortley Montagu, *Turkish Embassy Letters*, pp. 80–2.
91. DeKay, *Sketches of Turkey*, p. 111.
92. Nutton, 'Reception', pp. 232–4.
93. Adam Smith, *The Wealth of Nations*, pp. 9–12.
94. Mead, *Discourse on Plague*, p. 84; Bašeski, *Ljetopis 1749*–1804, pp. 6–7, 10.
95. Edward Said, *Orientalism*, pp. 14–15.

CHAPTER

4

MAGIC AND PLAGUE IN THE OTTOMAN EMPIRE

INTRODUCTION

Another key aspect to understanding Ottoman notions of plague is that treatise writers until Hamdan's 1838 reform frequently referred to magic or esoteric knowledge in a variety of forms to call on or channel the supernatural, or forces unintelligible to human logic, to alleviate human suffering or avoid death. Certainly, writers during the sixteenth and early seventeenth centuries, such as Bitlisi and Taşköprüzade, cited the time-worn formulas of Ahmad al-Buni (d. 1225) and other believers in the ritual use of Quranic verses, words, prayers and talismans in an attempt to secure divine intervention to save one from the disease.[1] Ahmed Efendi similarly advocated astral magic to ward off plague in the Ottoman court during the late seventeenth century.[2]

Recent historians of science and medicine, beginning with Frances Yates, have successfully demonstrated that magic was also an elastic, but continuing element in European history during the thirteenth to the eighteenth centuries.[3] In the English case, for example, treatise writers on magic, including such sub-areas as cabala, a form of mystical understanding of the world based on Hebrew and Biblical texts, names and prayers, as well as astrology, divinations, conjuring, necromancy and alchemy, were profoundly affected by human tragedies (for example, London's great plague of 1665, the 1666 London fire, the English Civil War) and the social and ideological consequences of Protestant confessionalism. Similarly, the formation of an early modern English body politic, based in part on an emerging sea-borne merchant economy and a print culture reflective of those interests, also brought about significant change in the way magic was formulated and marketed by scholastics to their home audiences. Magical ideas prominent during this time included the cabala and talismanic astral understanding of elements and symbols to affect celestial and earthly elements. Cabala and talismanic enthusiasts often promoted a humanistic reassessment of religious texts. These enthusiasts often deconstructed classical conceptions of the world as an earth-centred Ptolemaic universe and as a global Galenic balance of the humors and the elements. One can also see a profound thread of both cabalistic and talismanic understandings of the plague in sixteenth- to eighteenth-century English plague literature, a still largely unexamined area in the historical literature.[4]

This chapter will suggest that, by referencing the English case, one can find comparable Ottoman cabalistic and astrological understandings of plague throughout the early modern era. Arguably, Ottoman writers, such as Ahmed Efendi or the above-mentioned sixteenth-century Ottoman writers, had a world view that related in many ways to their English and European contemporaries. The question, however, is the extent to which these Ottoman writers' socioeconomic, cultural and geopolitical contexts, as reflected in their changing professions, audiences and markets, differentiated the function and content of their work from their English counterparts. A detailed analysis of Ottoman and English treatise literature as they relate to cabalistic and the talismanic/astrological understandings of plague is necessary to answer this question.

CABALISTIC UNDERSTANDINGS

The Ottomans

The sixteenth-century Ottoman treatises, such as those of Taşköprüzade and Bitlisi, use the 'knowledge of letters' (*ilmi-i huruf*) – a mystical understanding of the Quran, the names of God and prayers, through numbers, signs, symbols, elemental and astrological values attributed to the combination of the twenty-eight letters of the Arabic alphabet – to offer the reader a cure for plague. These formulas are, in all likelihood, traceable as far back as the eleventh-century work of the Islamic philosopher Ghazali.[5] Remarkably, Ghazali's, Taşköprüzade's and Bitlisi's work parallels the Jewish cabala, which developed alongside its Islamic contemporary not only in late medieval Andalusia, but in the succeeding centuries throughout the Mediterranean. Taşköprüzade, for instance, noted that he acquired a number of his formulas from Sephardic Jewish refugees to the Ottoman Empire after the Reconquista in 1492, who, allegedly after converting to Islam, passed on their knowledge to him.[6]

As in cabala, Ottoman practitioners of the knowledge of letters believed that they drew their energy from the intermediate plane of existence (*berza*) between the earthly and heavenly worlds. Humans, as a microcosm of the universe, were able to access all three of these worlds: the earthly in life; the heavenly in death; and the intermediate in one's dreams or imagination. Humans were especially vulnerable to the creatures of the intermediate plane: namely, angels, Satan and, most frequently, spirits, or *jinn*. *Jinn* were the most directly responsible for inflicting a human victim with the plague by stinging him with a spear or arrow. (Plague treatise writers most often used the term *taun* for 'plague', as another form of its three-letter Arabic root (*ta'n*), which is translated as 'spear' or 'arrow'.) Indirectly, Satan himself would lead the *jinn* to plague the people, as Bitlisi argues was the case during Muhammad's day when the plague left Medina and devastated the nearby town of Cahka. Azrail, the angel of death, took the soul of each victim from his or her body when and if the plague victim died.

The treatises offer an arsenal of names (*esma*), letters (*huruf*) and numbers (*ebced*) that one can use to get rid of the *jinn* when it appears. Often the prayers would cite one of the ninety-nine names of God, such as the Believer (*Mumin*), the Nearest (*Karib*), the Purest (*Safi*), the Venerator (*Receb*), the Strongest (*Kavi*), the Mighty (*Muktedi*), the Everlasting (*Baki*), the Destroyer (*Helak*) and the Universal Guardian (*Rakib*). Very frequently, the author would ask the user to repeat the name, or a similar religious word, a distinct number of times.[7] For instance, Taşköprüzade directed that:

> Reading the name 'the Everlasting' 136 times every day during a plague will save you from the attack of the jinn of a *taun*. Reading other names such as Islam 371 times will save oneself from *taun*. This prayer is so powerful that the person who says it will not be harmed even if they step on a scorpion.[8]

The number of times a name should be repeated could often refer to a three- or four-digit alphabetical number code, which only the initiate would have access to, the letters most often forming the three- or four-letter root of yet another name of God.

Many of the prayers would refer to these names in order to call on a celestial power. For example, Taşköprüzade stated that:

> Putting the name 'the Mighty' at the end of a Quran will save you from plague. This will effect the harvest moon in the East, which is connected to the planet Jupiter.[9]

Sa'deddin Süleyman bin Muhammed Emin Müstakimzade, a late eighteenth-century chronicler, gave similar prescriptions:

> In the first night of a lunar month (*gure*), one should mention a name 'the Everlasting' 341 times and touch his body with his hand to get rid of the hidden

disease [plague] . . . One can write also inscribe the name 'the Purest' on a pumpkin leaf, and put it into violet oil. Hang it on a tube (*şişe*) exposed to the Sun. The person should memorize the name 391 times per day. The oil should be diffused and used like a lotion to protect oneself against plague.[10]

Some of the texts even cross into the sphere of magic which combined cabalistic and talismanic elements. Taşköprüzade called for the writing of God's name on to a person's forehead, the place according to astral magicians where a person's celestial fate would be inscribed.[11] Müstakimzade stated that:

> The name of God 'Universal Guardian' (*Rakib*) should be written on to a blank sheet and place under a rock seal or should be written on a *miskal* of silver in order to ward off plague during one's life time. One can write the following on to a piece of paper (Arabic letters: *Elif*, *Lam*, *Re*, *Mim*, *Kaf*, *Kaf*, *Ye*, *Te*, *Be*, *Ded*, *Re*).[12]

The rock seal and sheet of silver were important as they connected the name to a terrestrial element.

There are also a number of other passages pointing out the intermediary world of dreams and fears. Taşköprüzade mentions that one cure was revealed to a fifteenth-century Arabic practitioner while asleep:

> A disciple of Seyyid Ali-Hamdani saw Hamza in his dreams. Hamza gave him a prayer to expel plague and added that if a person's son is struck by plague, a certain prayer should be written on his fingernails depending on the location of the plague boil. If the boil is on the right side of the body, the prayer should be written on the left hand finger nails and vice versa.[13]

This prayer writing apparently hoped to restore the individual's mystical humoral balance. Another of Taşköprüzade's stories directly relates to the fear of plague and how it could open the gate to the plague-carrying genies (*jinns*) from the intermediary world:

> During a plague in Kasgar, students saw shadows on the wall [of plague-carrying *jinns*]. They got scared because the creatures had arrows (*ta'n*) in their hands. The students were ordered to show paper with certain words to counter them. Those who had the paper were saved but those who did not perished.[14]

Despite the formulaic use of names, numbers and rituals to magically cure plague, the Ottoman plague treatise writers also emphasised that ultimately it was God who was responsible for turning the disease. Taşköprüzade reflected this tendency in the following prayer:

> We ask You to protect us from Your deep sorrow . . . O You who have complete power and total control, O You who have hidden kindness, save us from what we are afraid of. The name of God is the best name. He is the God of the earth and the sky. With the name of God nothing will hurt us, neither on earth nor in the sky. And He listens to us and knows everything . . . In the names of God, the All-Compassionate and All-Merciful, I am asking You. O God, O Believer (*Mumin*), O Protector (*Muheymen*), O Dear (*Aziz*), O All-Compelling (*Cebbar*), please rid us of plague . . . O God, You are All-Capable (*Muktedir*) and I am the result of that. You are the owner and I belong to You. You are strong and I am weak. You are rich and I am poor. There is no God but You. Everything will disappear except your kind face . . . By Your names, Your hidden kindness . . . [and] the number of Your words, please [give] us . . . a remedy.[15]

Here, one gains the sense that reading God's names, and comprehending their mystical, numerical, spiritual meanings would ultimately lead to union with the divine: 'Everything will disappear except Your kind face'. This would imply ascent into heaven, the celestial world. At the same time, however, Taşköprüzade was pleading to God for mercy from people's pain and suffering on earth: 'You are the source of recovery . . . please [give] us . . . a remedy'.[16]

The treatise made similar commentaries with regard to the Quranic verses they use in their ritual prayers. The most frequent set of verses to be cited in plague prayers, 'The Opening' (*Al-Fatihah*), the opening lines of the Quran, touches directly upon this theme of God as the remedy for human suffering:

> In the name of God, the Most Gracious, Most Merciful: Praise be to God, the Cherisher and Sustainer of the Worlds. The Most Gracious, Most Merciful. Master of the Day of Judgement. Thee do we worship, and Thine aid we seek.[17]

Another frequently cited verse is from 'The Throne Verse' (*Ayat al-Kursi*), which states in part: 'His are all things in the heavens and on earth; who is there that can intercede in His presence except as He permitteth?' One also finds the Quran's promise that: 'If God touches thee with affliction, none can remove it but He; and if He touches you with happiness, He hath power over all things.'[18]

The Ottoman plague treatises best illustrate such statements of dependence on God's grace coupled with the possibility of individual action through the use of the magical knowledge of letters in two specific prayers. The first, attributed to the great Sufi mystic Ghazali (d. 1111), but actually penned in the sixteenth century, is in fact part of a circular talisman of letters and alphabetical numbers that was intended for the beneficiary to wear around his or her neck. The prayer that was necessary to activate the talisman reads:

> To You, my God, I extended my palms in every hardship and I received Your grace from every direction. I do not hope from You anything that You are not part of. If I have gravely sinned, it is not hidden from You. You were kind in the past. You are capable of protection in every situation and from every consequence.[19]

The above statement is similar to the earlier prayers in that it calls for divine intervention to cure the disease. One does not find, however, any specific reference to the *jinn*, a genie or evil spirit that caused the calamity. Instead, the author raises the possibility that the prayer is invalid if being cured is not part of God's ultimate plan, such as when the victim is struck by plague as a punishment for his or her sins. Thus, the prayer reflects a sense of humility in that the victim does not know God's ultimate purpose even if armed with a reinvigorated mystical understanding of the divine.

One can see this humility even in the directions the author gives to reproduce the talisman. Those who reproduce it should be ritually clean, and aware of his or her duty of charity to the poor and those afflicted with disease or pain. 'God created every trouble', but it was the writer's duty to attempt to alleviate suffering.[20] An illustration of the actual circle, with the prayer above it (see Figure 4.1), is useful for considering the talisman's more magical functions.

The nineteen Arabic letters and numbers (including a remarkable number of ones and nines) correspond to a Quranic verse, which only the plague-bearing *jinn* that came upon the bearer of the talisman would be aware of. The letters also mystically combine into a variety of God's names: potentially far stronger than simply a single name. If the owner did not happen to don the talisman before being struck with the plague, he or she also had the option of drinking an elixir consisting of water poured on the circle. (At least one reader of the text may well have done so given the smudges and watermarks on the original).[21]

The second example is an oft-cited prayer from Taşköprüzade:

> The Name of God is the very kind and very great proof. God is the ruler and does whatever He wants to. There is no power or force but by God, the exalted and great. I take refuge in God from Satan the cursed with the name of God the All-Compassionate and All-Merciful. O God I take refuge in You from the spear (*ta'n*), the plague (*taun*), calamities, sudden death, from being lost in worldly affairs and from bad actions (*kaza*).[22]

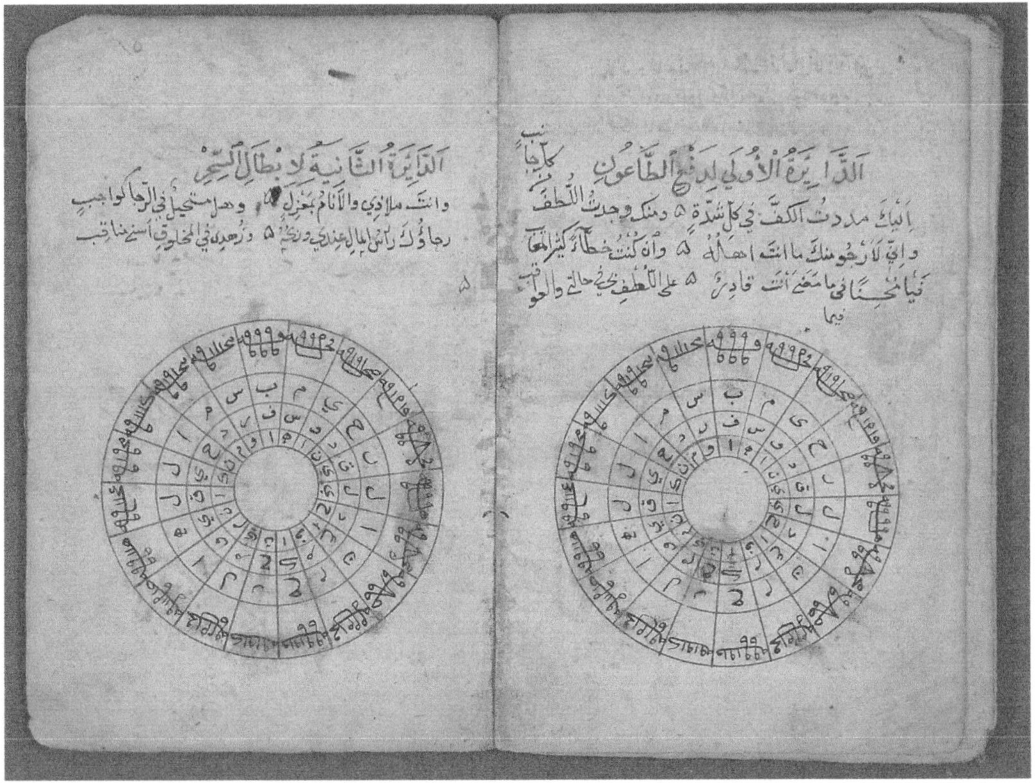

Figure 4.1 Ghazali's magical talisman

Source: Facsimile reprinted from Ebu Hamid Muhammed b. Muhammed Al-Gazali, *Cünnetü'l-Esmai'l-Mücerrebe li'l Vebai ve't-Taun*. Hacı Selimağa Library, Kemankeş 303 (undated), fols 16A–B, courtesy of Süleymaniye Library.

Here Taşköprüzade appears to limit his appeal and use of names directly to God, and connect the plague and the *jinn* who inflicted it to demonical forces. As in earlier passages, naming God was not mere human-initiated manipulation of celestial powers, but in fact mystical union with God. As formulated, this prayer asks God to either expel plague, or forgive the supplicant for a 'sudden death', 'being lost in worldly affairs' and from sins by welcoming him or her to the afterlife.

This passage is repeated three times in the text, surrounded by the formulas, names and numbers one is supposed to use in conjunction with the prayer, but there are also two significant variations. In one citation – inserted before the last sentence in the above version – it states:

> O God, the protector of kinship, drive plague away from us by the right of our Muhammad, the beloved elected one. God commend and salute Muhammad, his family, and friends.[23]

This statement implies that Muhammad, his family and companions may be able to intercede on behalf of the plague victims in a saint-like fashion.

A second variation reveals that Taşköprüzade was willing to speak to issues of fate and human interaction:

> O He who has all the glory and kindness (*ikram*). In name of God who is known as the great Lord. Every day He is in a different situation. What God wants to happen will happen, and what he does not want to happen will not happen. There is no power except the great exalted God.[24]

Here Taşköprüzade's statement parallels Ghazali's prayer in that he too seems to imply that the individual's fate is up to God's ultimate plans, and perhaps was a form of punishment or trial, rather than a wanton attack by a demon-inspired *jinn*. Regardless, one must conclude that both Taşköprüzade and the Ghazali texts reflect a great degree of flexibility in terms of spiritual and mystical function to combat the great human suffering and insecurity plague had inflicted upon their societies.

The English

Remarkably, English spiritual treatises about plague from the fifteenth to the seventeenth centuries strike a number of common themes with their Ottoman contemporaries. This similarity can be seen in prayers against the plague, on saintly intercession and on the use of divine names. Perhaps the most striking example of such similarities can be seen in Psalm 91, the single most frequently referenced biblical material in early modern English plague literature:

> [1] You who live in the shelter of the Most High who abide in the shadow of the Almighty [2] will say to the LORD, 'my refuge and my fortress; my God, in whom I trust'. [3] For he will deliver you from the snare of the fowler and from the deadly pestilence; [4] He will cover you with his pinions, and under his wings you will find refuge; his faithfulness is a shield and buckler. [5] You will not fear the terror of night, or the arrow that flies by day, [6] or the pestilence that stalks in darkness, or the destruction that wastes at noonday. [7] A thousand may fall at your side, ten thousand at your right hand, but it will not come near you. [8] You will only look with your eyes and see the punishment of the wicked. [9] Because you have made the LORD your refuge, the Most High your dwelling place [10] no evil shall befall you, no scourge come near your tent. [11] For He will command His angels concerning you to guard you in all your ways. [12] On their hands they will bear you up, so that you will not dash your foot against a stone. [13] You will tread on the lion and the adder; the young lion and the serpent you will trample underfoot. [14] Those who love me, I will deliver; I will protect those who know my name. [15] When they call to me, I will answer them; I will be with them in trouble, I will rescue them and honour them. [16] With long life will I satisfy them and show them my salvation.[25]

One sees the invocation of at least four of God's names (that is, the Most High, the Almighty, the Lord and my God). All four of these names had distinct references in their Hebrew original, paralleling the later Muslim use of the ninety-nine names of God. Moreover, the use of these names is highlighted in two formulas: 'He is my refuge and my fortress, my God, in whom I trust' (verse 2) and 'you have made the LORD your refuge' (verse 9). At least two prominent Biblical and Talmudic scholars have claimed that these are in fact formulaic phrases that guaranteed its user divine intervention.[26] As was seen in the Ottoman prayers, this intervention, 'gaining refuge in God', could mean either union with or deliverance from the plague.

Seemingly, however, the prayer guarantees deliverance from the disease itself. Interestingly, the Psalm, like the Ottoman prayers, makes a direct connection between plague and demonic forces. A number of scholars have traced phrases, such as 'the terror of night', 'the arrow that flies by day', 'the pestilence that stalks in the darkness' and 'the plague that destroys at midday' to specific names of demons from Babylonian and other ancient Middle Eastern mythologies, such as 'Lilth', the witch of the darkness, 'Namroth' and the Babylonian demon of pestilence. The prayer, originally written in the post-Babylonian exile period, also apparently has the common Middle Eastern imagery of a winged god.[27] Nevertheless, the text may also have reduced former gods like Lilth and Namroth to merely evil spirits, something very much akin, perhaps, to the *jinn* in Islamic sources. Over time, such imagery could also have had a great syncretic value for worshipers. One sees, for instance, that the Psalm mentions the role of angels as guardians in protecting the believer from plague. Thus, the supplicant appealed to one God for intervention, but allowed the possibility for another being, 'a servant of God' to intercede on His behalf.

At least some of the prayer's message (for example, the plague as arrows tied to evil spirits that required the name of God to get rid of it, a special prayer directed at God who alone understood the secret demonical cause of the plague) had a resonance among the spiritualist writers on plague. These included Henry Holland, a Calvinist preacher who wrote a commentary on Psalm 91 in 1593; William Kemp, who wrote a broader account on the causes (spiritual and otherwise) of the Great Plague that struck London in 1665; as well as E. Davies, whose sermon on plague was published shortly after the Marseilles outbreak in 1720.[28]

Other documents promised saintly intercession, such as a 1520 receipt that granted the bearer deliverance from plague in return for the donation of time or monies to the hospital of St Roche in Exeter:

> The graces following be granted to all brethren, sisters, benefactors and good-doers unto the hospital of the blessed confessor St. Roche founded and established within Lyte Exeter. If they do a Pater Noster, Ave Maria and the Crede it is granted them that they shall never be affected nor grieved with the stroke of pestilence. It more plainly appears in his legend how and when Almighty God granted to this petition to the said confessor St. Roche sent by his angel Raphael.[29]

Apparently, the belief that an intermediary of God, such as St Roche, and perhaps the angel Raphael, could save one from plague was common enough in England that it could be used as part of a pious foundation's market strategy.

The prayers to which the document alludes, namely, the Our Father, Hail Mary and the Nicene Creed, bear similar features to the above-cited plague prayers. While the Hail Mary prominently included a request for 'Mary, full of grace' to intercede on the believer's behalf and the Nicene Creed recognised God as the creator of the invisible (for example, spirits), the Our Father praised the name of God (that is, 'hallowed be Thy Name') in order to save the supplicant (that is, 'deliver us from evil'). The Our Father, in conformity with many such prayers, both Christian and Muslim, also implied that human suffering undoubtedly also resulted from sin (that is, 'lead us not into temptation').

One should finally note that such beliefs in the possibilities of divine intervention very well may have had a long-lasting symbolic legacy: the red cross, which was used by the English authorities in the mid-seventeenth century as the sign of a household or place struck by plague. The red cross, by no strange coincidence, was also tied to the myth of St Roche.[30] This patron saint of plague sufferers was born with the symbol of the red cross on his breast, and after a lifetime of service to the sick and needy, was popularly commemorated in England and Scotland in particular. The oft-used phrase 'Lord have mercy' also recalls the common themes of plague prayers, despite the fact that no outward published reference to the saint survived the Protestant-dominated London of 1665.[31]

Yet there were cries throughout the seventeenth century for a reformed understanding of the plague which was highly critical of ritualistic spiritual healing. James Balmford, writing after the plague outbreak in 1625, told his audience that material remedies were much more in order: '[Do] not . . . depend on extraordinary means (miracles and such like) when we may enjoy ordinary [ones].' At best, invoking plague prayers like Psalm 91 would be a vain attempt to understand God's secrets: 'For it is written . . . that secret things belong to God and revealed things belong to us.' At worst, using prayers to secure divine intervention would be 'tempting God' in a way similar to that of Satan in tempting Jesus to throw himself down from the top of the Jerusalem Temple knowing that God the Father would be obligated to save him.[32]

Unsurprisingly, there were cries by people like Thomas Hastler, who used similar arguments in 1615 to denounce earlier plague practices as heretical 'papism':

> But if it were possible for them to hear such unlawful prayers of men, they would with both hands (as we say) put them from them, and laboured to purge themselves from such flat idolatry, with their song of obedience. *Not onto us Lord, not onto us, but to thy name be such honour ascribed.*
>
> But our Romish doctors, to maintain their invocations of celestial spirits, do cozen simple people nowadays (as their predecessors did the Christians in the apostles' time) under the pretence of humility, saying that the God of all things was invisible, inaccessible and incomprehensible: and therefore (as Theodoret testifies) they counselled their followers to procure God's favour by the means of angels: like as the heathen idolaters to cover the shame of their neglecting of God . . . The very same rag our Romanists had borrowed from them to cover their superstition with that wickedness thereof might not appear.[33]

Here Hastler brands any type of prayer for intercession as akin to demonical witchcraft. Just as using God's name in such a prayer was sacrilege, as the name's honour belonged to God alone, so too calling on any intermediary, angel or saint alike, was heretical nonsense:

> Rome would have us believe that during the time of pestilence we must pray onto none but Saint Sebastian, and his successor, Saint Roche, saints invented to intercede against such a deadly disease: wilfully and directly opposing and contradicting the command and counsel of the Lord of Hosts.[34]

Stories of magic causing plague, rather than curing it, began to gain much more currency:

> In the year of Our Lord 1572 when a certain woman of Rezna in Poland was buried near the Church of the Exultation of the Holy Cross, the plague began to rage and spread extremely.[35]

The author of this passage, William Kemp, related another story from Simon Kelwaye in 1593 of ill-fated 'natural magic' as responsible for the troubles of his own times:

> When we see young children flock themselves together in companies, and then all will feign some of their company to be dead amongst them, and solemnise the burial in a mournful sort, this is a token which has been well observed in our age to foreshadow great mortality at hand . . . And I have heard that one did foretell our late unhappy civil wars, by seeing boys and children make officers, muster and imitate the train bands; saying, when he was in Germany, before the wars did there begin, the children there did the like.[36]

The question here, however, is what Kemp saw as the ultimate cause of the plague outbreak in 1665, and, by inference, the recent English Civil War. Did child play cause the plague or make their countrymen engage in open warfare or was the ultimate explanation to be found in imagination. The issue then would be, if the plague or wars started as a stray thought, would it be tied to the demon-ridden intermediary world or would it be instead the product of human imagination, a new-fangled microcosmic idea which would make man, not God, the focal point of disease and the universe at large.

Undoubtedly, writers like Henry Holland in 1593 still clung to the idea that demonic spirits caused plague, regardless of whether a ritualistic name-based spell could inflict or cure the disease:

> They [the plague-bearing evil spirits] persuade by a marvellous and invisible means, piercing by reason of their airy, thin bodies, the bodies of man when they perceive it not, and so confounding and mingling themselves by means of some imaginations conceived, with the motions of their minds both waking and sleeping.[37]

One does not perceive similar sentiments among the plague treatise writers by the time the plague struck London in 1665:

> The plague . . . is spread by fear and imagination. From the heart proceed the vital spirits, which are its lifeguard, and if they by fear are dissipated, or retire inwards, or leave the outward parts forsaken, which in infectious times are as it were environed and besieged with pestilential air, in comes the plague like a prevailing enemy, and easily enters the gates, scales the walls, and surprises the heart, which like a coward in extremity of danger, is not able to help itself, or make resistance.[38]

The above statement focuses on the concept of vital spirits, an idea originally coined by Aristotle, that a spirit or soul was the organising principle to the human body. What we see here, however, is a fundamental revision of that concept, in human-centred terms. Prior to the seventeenth century, God was ultimately responsible for determining a vital spirit's final cause. Now, we find, similar to Descartes' philosophy on mind and body, that the person could control their own health by controlling their emotions. Thus, if human rationality conquered fear, it could also conquer plague itself.[39] John Gadbury, an astrologist contemporary of William Kemp, confirmed this when he wrote of plague that:

> We find experimentally, that our reason and understanding, and all our noblest faculties, are led captive by our imagination *ad libitum*; and we are enslaved ignobly, and yet to remain such fools as to indulge our injurer.[40]

Others, like Thomas Brooks, a preacher who wrote a plague treatise shortly before he himself perished in the 1665 outbreak, took a far dimmer view of the human rational ability to overcome nature:

> The plague is more immediately from God, than any other sickness or disease; it is the immediate stroke of God. The scribe is more properly said to write than the pen; and he that make and keep the clock is more properly said to make it go and strike than the wheels and poizes that hang upon it: and every workman to effect his work rather than the tools which he used as instruments. So the Lord of Hosts, who is the chief Agent and Mover in all things, and in all actions, may more fitly and properly be said to effect and bring to pass all judgements, yea, all things which are done in the earth, than any inferior or subordinate causes; seeing they are but his tools and instruments, which He rules and guides according to His own will, power, and providence . . . Certainly, those are physicians of no value, that cannot look above second causes to the First Cause, they cannot

> look to *the wheel within the wheel.* The plague is a hidden thing, a secret thing; it is a sickness, a disease, but more immediately comes from God than any other sickness or disease does.[41]

Here Brooks posited that the plague's divine logic simply surpassed the physician's ability to overcome it. A key difference between Brook's vision and that of a number of earlier attributions of plague to a divine cause was not his despairing of divine salvation from death, but his mechanical vision of the God-driven order.[42] He used this vision, however, not to justify material measures against the disease, but to prove that such measures were indeed hopeless. This begged the question why an all-powerful God would use plague to kill good people:

> that some of the best of the Christians should fall by the pestilence, when many of the worst of sinners have their lives for a prey; these are some of those mysterious providences that many times make some of the best Christians to stagger in their judgement; and why so, but because they look upon God's proceedings through a double *medium* of flesh and spirit; hence it comes to pass all things seemed to run cross, and that God's most just and righteous proceedings, are not so clearly and fully discerned as might otherwise be. The wheels in a watch or in a clock move contrary to one another, some one way, some another, yet all show the skill and intent of the workman, to show the time, or to make the clock to strike: so in this world divine providence is seen to run cross to divine promises; the wicked are spared, and the righteous are taken away; yet in the conclusion all issues in the will, purpose and glory of God.[43]

Again, in contrast to Kemp and Gadbury,[44] Brooks offers no hope of either spiritual material or human initiative against the disease itself. God's logic was simply beyond mankind's comprehension, leaving the individual with the sole task of pursuing his or her understanding of God's ultimate justice. Curiously enough, Brooks uses cabalistic imagery to illustrate this point:

> I have read of a lodestone in Ethiopia, which has two corners, with the one that draws iron to it, with the other it puts the iron from it: so God has two arms, the one of mercy, and the other of judgement; two hands, the one of love, the other of wrath; with the one he draws, with the other he drives; the one strokes, the other strikes: and as he has a right hand of favour, wherewith leads to the saints, so he wants not a left hand of fury, wherewith to dash the wicked to pieces.[45]

This passage once again highlights Brooks' argument that God's power was embodied in material logic. A mere human being could not grasp the physical principle behind the logic, but it could understand its spiritual existence. The goal was, thus, to seek mystical union with the divine, with its implicit recognition of the Hebrew cabalistic stages of 'God's two arms': *Din*, 'judgement' or the arm of 'wrath'; and *Hesed*, 'mercy' or the arm of 'love'.[46] In contrast to understandings of the cabala as a multi-stage spiritual bonding in the present world, Brooks saw this pathway to salvation as lying only in death.

Brooks used a second, more talismanic illustration to make the same argument:

> Though death, through the pestilence, be to the wicked as the rod in Moses' hand that was turned into a serpent; yet to the godly, death, the pestilence, is like the wand in Elijah's hand, a means to waft them over into a better life.[47]

In his eyes, magic, like science, or even spiritual promises like Psalm 91, was limited to death and a promise of life after death. Nevertheless, it is striking how Brooks identified spiritual equality as yet another theme in this process:

> So 'tis here, the noisome pestilence, or the pestilence of grief (as the Hebrew runs in Psalm 91:3) has an equal aptness to cut down one man as well as another, the rich as well as the poor, the honourable as well as the base, the strong as well as the weak, the prince as well as the peasant, the emperor as well as the carter.[48]

This vision of death and the dispatch of the victim to eternal judgement as a great equaliser was matched by the positive vision of social utopia for those who reached heaven:

> The promises of God are a Christian's Magna Charta, his chief evidence that he has to show for his preservation, for his protection, for his salvation . . . O how highly do men prize their charters and privileges! And how carefully do they keep and lay up the conveyances and assurances of their lands! O how should then saints treasure up those precious promises, which are to them instead of all conveyances and assurances for their preservation, maintenance, deliverance, comfort, and everlasting happiness.[49]

This statement first implies that the quest for greater political and social equality may have also been a hopeless material endeavour. To Brooks, there was no sense in grasping 'charters and privileges' when the saintly plague victim could keep God's promise of eternal life. Oddly, Brooks also noted that such promises include Psalm 91's guarantee of divine deliverance from plague, when his passage infers that this may well simply be an earthly 'charter and privilege'.

Could it be that Brooks in despair is asking his readers to discard this 'promise' in the hope of ultimate redemption? If so, this would imply a problem with Psalm 91: was it the accurately recorded word of God? Could Brooks possibly have implied that the meaning of the scripture itself also defies human comprehension or that it was mistakenly recorded in the first place? Either interpretation would lead to questions about biblical authority that many Protestants of Brooks' day would certainly have taken issue with as it questioned the then cherished principle of *sola scriptura*.[50]

It is remarkable to note the pervasive sense of despair and fear in the English spiritual plague literature given the general argument that 'progressive' and 'effective' measures like quarantine and other state-initiated reform had alleviated human tragedy to a much greater extent than when the plague first broke out in 1347–8. One finds instead that both the writers and their audiences reflected the frustrations of their times. The seventeenth century may have allowed for a new mechanical philosophy that increasingly saw the individual and the state as being able to master nature and its calamities, but the reality was that tens of thousands of died of plague despite the quarantines and the Bills of Mortality. A wealth of new medical activity did nothing to stop the continued demand for a spiritual solution.[51]

The effect of confessionalist propaganda and the desire to control and discipline individual spiritual activity had only lessened the ability of the audience to resort to ritualistic prayer and saint worship. This can be seen most clearly not only in Hastler's anti-Catholic polemics, but also in the changing attitudes towards cabalistic prayers like Psalm 91. One can speculate that even in the early sixteenth century the common worshiper still had ready access to church-supported ritualistic prayers in the hope of saving oneself from plague, perhaps even including chants of God's names to secure divine intervention. But by 1593, with the rise of the Puritan movement and the consolidation of Elizabeth I's Protestant state, popular lay preachers like Henry Holland would avoid interpreting Psalm 91 as a cabalistic formula, even though he would maintain the belief that the prayer – as a reflection of God's will – could still save one from the plague. By 1665, even this deterministic faith in God's grace would give way to others who either despaired of spiritual solutions or turned to the new-found belief that human emotions determined who lived and who died from plague.

Certainly, there are significant comparisons to be made between Ottoman and English cabalistic perceptions. Admittedly, there are definite similarities in approach between the two bodies of narrative accounts. The letter magic, the names of God, ritualistic prayer, the stress on the divine and the possibility of saintly and even human initiated salvation from plague that one found in Taşköprüzade, Bitlisi and the Ottoman version of Ghazali's circle found a correspondence in similar patterns in Psalm 91 and the lasting popularity of St Roche.[52] The differences were not to be found in religious content, but rather the social and economic context of the early modern era. The rapid rise of an overseas merchant-based economy in the booming city of London resulted in fundamental changes in the purpose and audience of the spiritual plague treatise writers. While earlier writers were tied to the relatively limited circles of courts, and literate and religious elites and had a relatively small circulation, the late sixteenth- and early seventeenth-century English writers expanded their message via print to new urban and commercial audiences.[53] This exposed the writers to state-driven concerns of religious orthodoxy, suppressing religious dissent and, as seen in Brooks, calls for the meek acceptance of one's fate.

The transformation of magical imagery is perhaps the best example of this trend. Whereas magic was practised by religious elites and commoners alike prior to the late sixteenth century, the use of cabalistic chants was increasingly restricted thereafter. Seemingly, the only ones who could use such concepts were those literary and religious elites who applied it ideologically to justify an array of reforms or social disciplinary ideas. Brooks's symbolic use of the Jewish cabala, Moses' and Aaron's magic rod and wands, like that of the divine watch-maker metaphor are clear examples of this trend. His symbols conveyed the message of accepting one's fate and limiting social dissatisfaction in a time of grief and dismay. Such imagery, like the preceding propaganda of religious and social intolerance, was a dark aspect of early modern history that the Ottomans simply did not have to deal with.

ASTROLOGY AND TALISMANIC UNDERSTANDINGS OF PLAGUE

The Ottomans

Ahmed Efendi's composition of an treatise on astrology and the plague in the mid- to late seventeenth century provides a great number of insights into changes within astrological practice in the Ottoman Empire during this time and the increasing role of talismanic magic. Earlier texts, such as Bitlisi and Al-Yahudi, acknowledged celestial causes as the reason behind plague, citing Quranic or ancient philosophical texts as their prime authorities. Bitlisi, for example, argued that the Quran states that 'day came into existence with the rising of the sun' and that God created plants and animals in alignment with celestial bodies: 'Every piece of earth is tied to the heavens. The heavens have power over those subordinate to it.'[54] This was perhaps best demonstrated by the continual effect of the sun and moon on tides and the earthly environment:

> Celestial bodies like the sun, the moon and stars can cause putrefication as well as health. For example, if the moon does not cool, then seas and rivers will shrink as a result, and herbs and trees will die from thirst.[55]

Al-Yahudi argued that Plato and Hippocrates had shown that the conjunction of Mars and Saturn was responsible for triggering plague. Al-Yahudi further posited that such celestial movements caused earthquakes, storms and other elemental eruptions that would lead to the creation of plague-bearing miasmas. While Al-Yahudi and Bitlisi prescribed various material measures, and Bitlisi also advocated prayer and enumerating the cabalistic names of God, none of these authors saw any elemental, or talismanic magic that could be used to alleviate this situation.[56]

In contrast, Ahmed Efendi made a fundamentally different argument. He emphasised the importance of mastering the strange magical connection between the elements, individual human beings and the stars beyond to understand, prevent and cure the plague. He claimed that gaining an accurate reading of one's horoscope, including the ascendant sign that a person has at his or her birth, was critical to learning the nature of this connection. An astrologer like him would understand one's 'ascendancy by looking at a person's eyebrows'. Consequently, after looking at the individual's horoscope he could, with knowledge of the secret ore for each ascendant star, cast a mould figure of the individual to ward off plague. The mould figure would be made of a certain metal (for example, copper if the person's ascendant star was Venus or tin if Jupiter) and might bear the secret name of a spirit or shape. If that person had the misfortune to be born under an unlucky star, he could 'turn a bad sign into a good one by using certain intoxicating elements like opium'. Such talismans were compounds of terrestrial and celestial bodies that solved a problem.

Similar talismans could be produced for affecting a city or region; For example, jade was known for causing rain. A brass talisman of a snake was forged and placed at the hippodrome in Istanbul to ward off snakes. Spells were also to be used, either in conjunction with the talismans or independently. Ahmed Efendi related the story of how Caliph Memun used a spell to get rid of all the beetles in Baghdad, and how another used a similar incantation to clear Damascus of its scorpions, mice, snakes and spiders.[57]

Three further aspects of Ahmed Efendi's work needs to be highlighted in particular. First, his work on magic, in contrast to Bitlisi and the Ottoman advocates of the 'knowledge of letters', does not refer to magic's tie to the divine, or even to earlier ancient Greek or medieval Arab scholars. This is notable given the traditional citation in these works to Quranic and/or scholastic sources. Curiously enough, Ahmed Efendi was trained as a Mevlevi shaykh as well as an astrologer, and spent considerable time as a religious scholar in Mecca, Medina and Cairo after losing his post as the sultan's chief astrologer.[58]

Secondly, Ahmed Efendi's work reveals strategies that were typical of astrologers of that time. He clearly sought to use his book to regain the coveted post of court astrologer. While he gave a general introduction to his art in order to demonstrate his qualifications for that post – highlighting at least two earlier books he had written on the topic – he did not reveal any specific spells or details that others could use to secure the position instead.[59]

Finally, Ahmed Efendi seemed to be well aware of current trends within astrological practice. Not only did he spend time learning in the scholarly and religious centres of the Mediterranean Islamic world – he wrote his two books in Egypt and in Arabic – but he also hinted at an openness towards other more trans-regional trends, such as his mention of magic as being related to 'mathematics either unleashed from the power of geometry, or from the science of dynamics as seen in a pendulum'.[60] This could be an allusion to new trends that were popular among seventeenth-century scientific circles in Europe, and perhaps beyond.

The intercultural exchange of ideas was a two-way street, however. Raffael Gaffarel, a Frenchman who wrote a defence of astral magic translated into English in 1653, clarified that much of his inspiration on the use of talismans, spells and celestial powers was based on past and present Islamic practices. For example, Gaffarel claimed that the word 'talisman' was originally an Arabic word, and that some of the great Islamic scholars of medieval times, such as Almansor, Messahala, Zahel and Albohazen, were some of talismanic magic's most influential advocates. In Gaffarel's eyes, the Islamic symbol of the crescent and the Quranic story that the fallen angels Arot and Marot brought the knowledge of talismans with them when they travelled to earth, were other examples of this legacy.[61] Recent scholars of Islamic history, like T. Fahr, confirm that such influences were essential the revitalisation of talismanic magic by late sixteenth- and seventeenth-century intellectuals like Giordano Bruno and Gaffarel.[62]

Yet Gaffarel was undoubtedly aware of more recent talismanic practices in the Middle East. Interestingly, Gaffarel highlighted the use of talismans not only on ships to protect them from bad weather and in fields to insure good crops, but also in imperial cities like the former Byzantine capital of Constantinople. One such story, taken from the late Byzantine historian Doukakis, relates the use of a talisman to ward off insects:

> It is also reported, that after that Mahomet the Second had possessed himself of Constantinople, the breaking of the lower jaw of a brazen serpent was the cause of the increasing of serpents in those parts. So true it is, that these talismans have the power to direct many of those calamities that afflict mankind.[63]

Gaffarel's story tends to romanticise the Byzantines as somehow in tune with their talismanic, Greek past far more than their Ottoman successors, implying as many humanist scholars did that the transfer of ancient knowledge by Byzantine exiles was critical to the revitalisation of Europe's arts and sciences. One should note that this is in contrast to Ahmed Efendi's version of the story, which implies the Ottomans themselves cast the bronze talisman.[64]

Gaffarel pointed out a second, similar account that relates to the Byzantine talismanic practice against plague:

> At Byzantium, which is now Constantinople, there were many of these talismanic figures to be seen: but the fury of war has demolished them all, to the great prejudice of the inhabitants. Sultan Mahumet also caused one of them to be broken to pieces, which was a brazen horse, with a horseman upon him; which is certainly reported to have preserved the city from pestilence, and all contagion of the air: but since that time, this disease has raged so fiercely, as that in the space of four months, Leunclavius, who was present, affirms that there died 150,000 persons: and every year, in the months of July, and August, the like effect.[65]

This version once again reaffirms the idea that the Ottomans, particularly Sultan Mehmed II, failed to continue the valuable Byzantine practice of talismanic magic, to the detriment of Istanbul's population. Unsurprisingly, the account propagates the Byzantine version of the conquest of the city as the fall of a great civilisation to barbarism. The claim that Mehmed II destroyed an equestrian statue is significant given that Muslims detested images as symbols of ancient Greek and Roman greatness in the arts.

Nonetheless, one should also compare this account to that of Evliya Çelebi, the famous mid-seventeenth-century Ottoman traveller, who related yet another version. He claims that it was Mehmed II's son Bayazid II, a pious Muslim, who, during the construction of a series of new mosques in the old Byzantine city centre, tore down an ancient pillar erected by the Byzantines to commemorate the conversion to Christianity of the founder of the city, Emperor Constantine. According to Evliya, Bayazid quickly rebuilt the column after plague suddenly struck the city and killed his son.[66]

While Evliya's tale confirms that Bayazid, like Mehmed II, was initially ignorant of the value of talismans to protect the city from plague, it is significant that Bayazid actually rebuilt the column after learning a painful lesson.[67] Moreover, Evliya's inference that such talismans were used by the Ottoman rulers in Istanbul is confirmed by the survival of three such talismans in the middle of the hippodrome, the great parade ground of the city in both Ottoman and Byzantine times. There one can still find the bronze serpent, a smaller column and an Egyptian obelisk, all three talismanical objects that were dutifully maintained by the Ottomans, as is evident from the walls that they built around them. Constantine's monument, some half a kilometre away, similarly still stands today.

Also striking is Evliya's implication of a possible religious motivation for Bayazid, since Bayazid was known as a far more sincere Muslim than his father. Presumably, initially Bayazid could have torn down the column to symbolise his religion's ultimate conquest of Byzantine Christian civilisation. This part of the story corresponds with the earlier efforts of Byzantine authors and European travellers to build up the myth of Mehmed II as an intolerant barbarian. Some Ottoman chroniclers and Western travellers bolstered this claim, alleging that both Mehmed II and Bayazid II sought to rename the city as 'Islam-bol' or the 'full of Islam' rather than simply 'Istanbul', an Ottoman Turkish translation of 'Constantinople' that remains related to its original place name.[68] Evliya seemingly revised the myth in favour of a sultan who learned that the talisman's magical powers, and perhaps his own tolerance of his realm's Christian minority, was critical to his empire's survival and prosperity. Could it be that Evliya actually was using this story in a similar way to the alchemists of neighbouring European states who employed metaphors to justify ideas of tolerance in age of confessionalist war?[69]

The English

Evidence of such imagery is particularly clear in the dedications of the English treatise writers. For example, William Kemp started out with the following commemoration to his patron:

> To the King's most excellent Majesty Charles the Second, by the grace of God, King of England, Scotland, France, and Ireland; Defender of the Faith, etc.
>
> Most dread and gracious Sovereign: the glorious sun, who communicates his beams and light, not only to the stars and heavens where he doth reside, but also to the air and water, and the remotest part of the earth, where the lowest shrubs are cherished with his influence, is a fit emblem of your Majesty whose pious care was expressed not only for the nobles and courtiers, that have the honour to be near your person; but also for the Commons and inferior people, that have the happiness to be in your mind, in appointing and accepting the directions of the learned College of London, for the cure of, and preservation from the pestilence.[70]

This statement, very much reminiscent of Louis XIV (1638–1715), the 'Sun King' Charles II (1630–85) so very much admired, used the astrological symbol of the sun in the heavens to justify his rule in both earthly and celestial terms. Such symbols were an attempt to displace the earlier idea of divine right, which would imply the monarch's dependence on ecclesiastical authority, in favour of the natural legal notion that the universe, like the earth, was subject to lay rules and rulers. Such ideas appealed to kings and the war-torn populace alike, and helped to set in motion support for 'enlightened absolutist' rule.[71] There are no similar dedications in Ahmed Efendi's or the later Ottoman plague treatises, which leads me to believe that Evliya's symbolism and Ahmed Efendi's awareness of international trends in literature on astral magic were not due to patronage of ideological images from the court *per se*.

Another issue that Ottoman practitioners of talismanic magic did not have to deal with was the charge of heresy. Gaffarel's treatise was the only printed work in the English language that I found that attested to the use of talismans against plague, referring to the accomplishments of Paracelsus and Crollius, both controversial authors in the mid-seventeenth century:

> Now of late many learned men have rescued from oblivion these figures [talismans]; and Paracelsus did take so much pains herein, as that he made diverse of them; and those of such virtue, as that they preserved those that wore them from the pestilence, as many in Germany have had experience of . . . Those also which Paracelsus calls Zenexton, by a Made Name (it being the custom of this author, to devise new words), are made with exceedingly great art. In one of them there is a scorpion and a serpent figured: and he says it must be made when the sun and the moon enter into the sign of Scorpio. In another you have a great number of little holes, with in an oval. You may see the figures of them, in the chemical works of Crollius.[72]

Gaffarel then went on to note that Crollius faced charges of witchcraft for promoting such work. This pressure against occultist and talismanic magic led Gaffarel into an extended discussion as to why talismans actually confirmed acceptable Christian norms. For instance, he claimed that the art first emerged in ancient Israel. He offered discoveries such as the original Hebrew names for the planets (Jacob's son Gad being the name for the planet Jupiter), Moses' practice of the art and the sight of Hebrew letters in the heavens as proof in this regard. Only later, Gaffarel maintained, did the Egyptians corrupt talismanic magic.[73] He and other apologists for a Christian hermeticism, or talismanic magic, like Cornelius Agrippa, sought to restore the profession to what it once was.[74]

The English astrologers were far more sceptical of such speculation. As a whole they tended to defend their profession as a science as distinct from 'superstition', a category which implied talismanic magic. John Gadbury and William Lilly, two of the most prominent astrologists of the second half of the seventeenth century, wrote almanacs that used such astrological reasonings – minus talismans, spells and other magical components – to predict events from plagues to wars, and the lives of individual monarchs. Recognising the twelve zodiacs and the principles of ascendancy, they always argued their works to be the result of long labour over charts, together with foresight and the most modern knowledge of celestial movements scholars could provide.[75] Almanacs proved to be among the most popular books of their day, tending to have the highest circulation of any printed book short of the Bible during the seventeenth century.[76]

In fact, Lilly and Gadbury went so far as to maintain that astrology could prove plague's celestial causation of ineffectual miasmas rather than the contagionist argument popular among many physicians, particularly magistrates, members of the Royal Medical Society, and opponents of the Levantine cotton trade. At first, Lilly indirectly criticised such opinion in 1644, when he related how ineffectual the Habsburg College of Physicians were in accepting both a contagionist and an astrological cause for plague in 1599.[77]

Gadbury made the bold argument in the immediate aftermath of 1665 outbreak that the London Bills of Mortality proved that the plague waxed and waned according to the celestial movements of Saturn and Mars.[78] Oldenburg, chief of the Royal Medical Society, strenuously objected to Gadbury's support for the anti-contagionist camp in his correspondence with others like John Boyle.[79] John Graunt, whose work was central to the newly developing field of 'political arithmetic', also discounted such ideas in press in favour of contagionism.[80] Gadbury responded at length to a similar critique by a contemporary of Oldenburg and Graunt:

> There is another gentleman also, a doctor of physick (which title (fairly obtained) and possession of also, I exceedingly honour) has been pulling at me in print, for my maintaining the negative in the question above propounded. This antagonist is angry in earnest and tells the world that I deserve to be answered by the magistrate, and that there is no way to suppress my opinion, or answer my arguments, but by putting in execution an order published in Queen Elizabeth's days . . .
>
> And considering some other passages of his, I perceive that he is not more angry at that my opinion, than at the celestial movers, the stars; whom (he says) many have accused as the authors of plague. I have (I acknowledge) in the book before mentioned, proved the stars to be (Sub Deo) the causes of the pestilence.
>
> But this gentleman (not withstanding his aim, and fruitless pains, to render me ridiculous and the stars (I study) ineffacious;) is not (in the meantime) aware,

of his own running into an error of far greater magnitude; viz. in his asserting the original of the plague to have been ROTTEN MUTTON eaten in the year before.

Now let any rational man consider whether he comes nearest the truth; I, in asserting the stars; or he, in maintaining a rotten mutton, to be the cause of the pestilence. An epicurean may, and frequently does, ascribe more to his belly than on to those glorious and ever-busied lamps of heaven. I cannot stand here to repeat the arguments I have urged to prove the plague contagious; I must refer the reader, for that, to the book itself.

But if rotten mutton be attended with such fatal effects, why not a plague every year after a rot of sheep which is the consequence of every moist summer? Or, if the plague were truly the effect of rotten mutton; how else then does it hold true, what he asserts elsewhere, in the same discourse that the plague came from the Netherlands, and to them from Smyrna, in a parcel of infected goods? Was there a rotten mutton in Smyrna too?

To conclude: let us suffice at present, that I deny any such a way of infection by goods; and reject romance of his rotten mutton: and (as before) do assert, the stars (Sub Deo) to be the true and essential causes of all plagues.[81]

The jocular yet convincing tone of Gadbury's statement was central to convincing his audience to support the idea that celestial movements, not rotten mutton or imported Ottoman cotton, caused plague. This was likely to coalesce with the other anti-contagionist arguments that emphasised that imported goods – like lamb from the countryside or cotton from abroad – were far more of an economic benefit than a public health hazard. This undoubtedly appealed to Gadbury's mainstay: London's entrepreneurs. Gadbury went so far as to name his political opponents – a doctor pushing Elizabeth I's laws – and use the Bills of Mortality against them![82] It should be noted that Elizabeth I and her mercantilist advisers were the first to ban an import (French wine) in order to prevent the plague, much to the chagrin of the very shopkeepers Gadbury to whom would later appeal.[83]

Gadbury's combination of astrology and the Bills of Mortality also seem remarkably similar to the way in which practitioners of the cabalistic, occultist and talismanic arts, such as Marsilio Ficino, Pico della Miranda, Cornelius Agrippa and Giordano Bruno, justified the findings of Galileo. This proved once again that combinations of magic and scientific innovation readily sold to a body politic that sought to justify socioeconomic and geopolitical change.[84]

Moreover, Gadbury's work also illustrates a stark difference between Ottoman and English astrological literature. The English literature was aimed at a broad, politically and commercially active audience. Gadbury, Lilly and Kemp were much more in tune with the politics of state-building movements, which would justify absolutist notions of sovereignty, governmental regulation of religious and social affairs, and an emerging commercial economy. Astrological charts and tables that graphically illustrated the rise and fall of monarchs, the capturing of new markets, the founding of colonies and the outbreaks of disease tapped into this dynamic medium. One can almost imagine that Gadbury's pamphlets were as dog-eared as any recent publication in the coffee houses, libraries and homes of London at the time.[85]

Ottoman astrologers were certainly not totally isolated from such developments, as seen in Ahmed Efendi's and Gaffarel's shared talismanic magic, as well as Evliya's symbol of Bayazid's magical unification of the empire. However, Ottoman astrologers like Ahmed Efendi still worked within a court culture where their writings had a much smaller circulation. One should not overlook the fact that I have located only one new astrological tract in Ottoman Turkish on plague during the entire seventeenth century; a trend which contrasts strongly with the wealth of printed English astrological literature on plague during the same era.

While Ahmed Efendi and other Ottoman astrologists undoubtedly had an impact on the sultan and his family, palace intrigues and patronage, they did not play the same public, commercial role as London's treatise writers. Consequently, the Ottoman writers were not subject to the same type of ideological scrutiny as their English counterparts.

Gadbury's exclaimer at the beginning of his argument with the doctor that astrology was the superior cause of plague 'sub deo', or 'outside an act of God', was not there by mere accident.[86] This exception, like his and his colleagues' avoidance of talismanic elements in his astrological predictions, was a direct result of the confessionalist pressure to root out magical practices outside ideological images and justifications. Talismanic magic, like all cabalistic medicine and saint worship, allowed for a type of individual initiative and economy that the state and religious authorities would not allow in print.

CONCLUSION

The impact of print culture and the political, religious and commercial developments in London during the late sixteenth and seventeenth centuries help to explain why English and Ottoman plague treatises developed fundamentally different functions during this time. Even by the early sixteenth century, it appears that both the English and Ottomans had similar cabalistic perceptions and practices regarding plague in both courtly circles and on a more popular level. This is indeed a far cry from Dols' still dominant interpretation of the Ottoman's static mystical essentialist conceptions of plague.[87] Moreover, the religious authorities of the time also seemed to have sanctioned such practices. Although the English crown and new Protestant ecclesiastical authorities increasingly pressured such practices, particularly on a popular level, intellectual elites continued to cultivate the cabalistic and hermetic/talismanic arts for a much longer period. Ottoman intellectuals, represented by the likes of Ahmed Efendi and Evliya, likely remained in touch with these same schools of thought.

England's state and commercial formation, religious strife, civil war and natural disasters like the plague and the fire of London, put pressures on astrological and spiritual treatise writers on plague to act as ideological agents. Brooks' use of multilayered divine magical, cabalistic talismanic and even mechanical symbols of utopia in the world beyond; Gadbury's combination of astrology and the bills of mortality; as well as Kemp's dedication to Charles II as the 'Sun King', undoubtedly provided valuable justifications for English authorities overwhelmed by the crisis of 1665: social resignation to death from plague; faith that sciences like astrology would master epidemic disaster; and the belief in the sovereign as the source of earthly and celestial authority.

These works were simply state-encouraged efforts at social and political damage control rather than signs of progress against the ravages of pestilence. Undoubtedly, London's suffering masses were frustrated that the plague devastated the city regardless of the promises that quarantines and other medical regulations could contain the damage. References to natural magic, fear and imagination, as well as a growing disbelief that any preventive measure could alleviate the danger, reveal a sense of despondency to which only those who had suffered the untold horrors of religious and civil war could relate. The Ottomans, who remained outside such state-building movements, mechanical and social disciplinary ideologies, never had to 'spin' their way out of such a public accounting. Similar pressure would come about only towards the end of the eighteenth century, when the Europeans began to threaten the Ottoman social order in the name of a disease they had only imagined themselves to conquer.

NOTES

1. Bitlisi, *Hısn ül-veba*, fols 17A–25B, 33A, 73A–B; Dols, *The Black Death in the Middle East*, pp. 3–12, 281–302; Taşköprüzade, *Risale fi't-Taun ve'l-Veba*, fols 182A–5B, 188A.
2. Ahmed, *Risale fi İlmi Tılsım ve Def'i''t-Taun*.
3. Frances Yates, *Giordano Bruno and the Hermetic Tradition*, pp. 1–156; Frances Yates, *The Occult Philosophy in the Elizabethan Age*, pp. 3–4, 18–24, 35–46, 107, 116–24.
4. Balmford, *A Short Dialogue concerning the Plague's Infection*; Thomas Brooks, *A Heavenly Cordial for all those Servants of the Lord that have had the Plague . . ., or, Thirteen Divine Maximes, or Conclusions, in Respect of the Pestilence: Which may be as so Many Supports, Comforts and Refreshing Springs, both to the Visited and Preserved*

People of God in this Present Day: Also Ten Arguments to Prove that in Times of Common Calamity the People of God do stand upon the Advantage Ground as to their Outward Preservation and Protection . . .: Also Eight Reasons why some of the Precious Servants of the Lord have fallen by the Pestilence in this Day of the Lord's Anger; Thomas Hastler, *An Antidote against the Plague. Or Panchrestōn: A Salve for All Sores: which applied and practised, will soone awaken the Lord's Mercy, and suddenly cause the Storms of his Iust Judgements to vanish away. Delivered in a Sermon, preached within the Cathedrall Church of Saint Paules, London*; Henry Holland, *Spirituall Preseruatiues against the Pestilence: Or a Treatise containing Sundrie Questions: Both Concerning the Causes of the Pestilence, (Where is Shewed, that the Plague is a Mixt Euill of Knowne and Secret Causes, and therefore so Hardly Healed by Naturall Curatiues only) and the Most Pretious Preseruatiues against the Same and Many Other Euils. Chiefely Collected out of the 91 Psalme*; William Kemp, *A Brief Treatise of the Nature, Causes, Signes, Preservation from, and Cure of the Pestilence.*

5. Al-Ghazali, Ebu Hamid Muhammed b. Muhammed, *Cünnetü'l-Esmai'l-Mücerrebe li'l Vebai Ve't-Taun*, fols 4A–8A, 16A–18B.
6. Taşköprüzade, *Risale fi't-Taun ve'l-Veba*, fol. 188A.
7. Bitlisi, *Hısn ül-veba* fols 17A–25A, 33A, 73A–B; Taşköprüzade, *Risale fi't-Taun ve'l-Veba*, fol. 185B.
8. Taşköprüzade, *Risale fi't-Taun ve'l-Veba*, fols 182A–185B.
9. Taşköprüzade, *Risale fi't-Taun ve'l-Veba*, fol. 183B.
10. Müstakimzade, *Cihazü'l-Macun fi'l-Halas Mine't-Taun*, fol. 46B.
11. Taşköprüzade, *Risale fi't-Taun ve'l-Veba*, fol. 183A.
12. Müstakimzade, *Cihazü'l-Macun fi'l-Halas Mine't-Taun*, fol. 46A.
13. Taşköprüzade, *Risale fi't-Taun ve'l-Veba*, fol. 191B.
14. Taşköprüzade, *Risale fi't-Taun ve'l-Veba*, fol. 188B.
15. Taşköprüzade, *Risale fi't-Taun ve'l-Veba*, fols 184A–186B. I wish to thank Mohamed Ben Yahia for so kindly translating this and the following of Taşköprüzade's plague prayers in this chapter from Arabic to English.
16. Taşköprüzade, *Risale fi't-Taun ve'l-Veba*, fol. 187A.
17. Yusuf Ali Abdullah, *The Meaning of the Holy Quran*, pp. 14–15.
18. Abdullah, *The Meaning of the Holy Quran*, pp. 105, 247.
19. Al-Ghazali, *Cünnetü'l-Esmai'l-Mücerrebe li'l Vebai Ve't-Taun*, fol. 16 A.
20. Al-Ghazali, *Cünnetü'l-Esmai'l-Mücerrebe li'l Vebai Ve't-Taun*, fols 7A–B, 13A–B.
21. Al-Ghazali, *Cünnetü'l-Esmai'l-Mücerrebe li'l Vebai Ve't-Taun*, fol. 16A.
22. Taşköprüzade, *Risale fi't-Taun ve'l-Veba*, fols 187A, 188A.
23. Taşköprüzade, *Risale fi't-Taun ve'l-Veba*, fol. 187B.
24. Taşköprüzade, *Risale fi't-Taun ve'l-Veba*, fol. 188A.
25. Bruce Metzger et al., *The New Oxford Annotated Bible with the Apocrypha: An Ecumenical Study Bible Completely Revised and Enlarged*, pp. 753–4.
26. Walter Russell Bowie *et al.*, *The Interpreter's Bible*, vol. 4, pp. 493–7; J. J. Stewart Perowne, *The Book of the Psalms: A New Translation with the Introductions and Notes Explanatory and Critical*, vol. 2, pp. 493–6.
27. A. A. Anderson, *The Book of Psalms*, vol. 2, pp. 655–60; Othmar Keel, *The Symbolism of the Biblical World, in Ancient Near Eastern Iconography, and the Book of Psalms*, pp. 82–7, 97, 136, 180–1, 190–1, 223–5, 352–3.
28. E. Davies, *A Sermon Preach'd on Friday Decemb. 16th 1720 Being the Day of Publick*

Fasting and Humiliation for the Averting God's Judgments, particularly the Plague, pp. 4, 9–10; Holland, *Spirituall Preseruatiues against the Pestilence*, pp. 15–19, 34; Kemp, *A Brief Treatise* pp. 7, 10.

29. Anonymous, *The Graces Folowying be Graunted* . . . 1520.
30. Anonymous, *The Mourning Cross, or Lord Have Mercy upon us* . . . .
31. J. Campbell, 'Saint Roche', *New Catholic Encyclopedia*, vol. 12, pp. 540–1; Dols, *The Black Death in the Middle East*, p. 137, fn. 63.
32. Balmford, *A Short Dialogue concerning the Plague's Infection*, pp. 33, 60–2.
33. Hastler, *An Antidote against the Plague*, pp. 31–2, emphasis in original.
34. Hastler, *An Antidote against the Plague*, p. 21.
35. Kemp, *A Brief Treatise*, p. 9.
36. Kemp, *A Brief Treatise*, p. 28.
37. Holland, *Spirituall Preseruatiues against the Pestilence*, p. 31.
38. Kemp, *A Brief Treatise*, p. 22.
39. Lex Newman, 'Epistemology of René Descartes', *Stanford Encyclopedia of Philosophy* (online edition).
40. John Gadbury, *London's Deliverance Predicted in a Short Discourse Shewing the Cause of Plagues in General, and the Probable Time (God Not Contradicting the Course of Second Causes) When the Present Pest May Abate, &c*, p. 27.
41. Brooks, *A Heavenly Cordial*, pp. 2–3, emphasis in original.
42. Davies, *A Sermon Preach'd on Friday Decemb. 16th* 1720, pp. 9–10.
43. Brooks, *A Heavenly Cordial*, pp. 61–2, emphasis in original.
44. Gadbury, *London's Deliverance*, p. 27; Kemp, *A Brief Treatise*, pp. 7, 10, 28.
45. Brooks, *A Heavenly Cordial*, pp. 74–5.
46. Danniel Matt, *The Essential Kabbalah: The Heart of Jewish Mysticism*, pp. 8–9.
47. Brooks, *A Heavenly Cordial*, p. 70.
48. Brooks, *A Heavenly Cordial*, p. 5.
49. Brooks, *A Heavenly Cordial*, pp. 19–20.
50. John Merriman, *A History of Modern Europe: From Renaissance to Present*, p. 132.
51. A. Lloyd Moote and Dorothy C. Moote, *The Great Plague: The Story of London's Most Deadly Year*, pp. 183–90.
52. Anonymous, *Graces*.
53. Elizabeth L. Eisenstein, *The Printing Revolution in Early Modern Europe*, pp. 3–91.
54. Bitlisi, *Hısn ül-veba*, fol. 29A.
55. Bitlisi, *Hısn ül-veba*, fols 70A–B.
56. Al-Yahudi, *Micennetü't-Ta'un ve'l-Veba*, fols 1A–30A; Bitlisi, *Hısn ül-veba*, fols 2A–79B.
57. Ahmed, *Risale fi İlmi Tılsım ve Def'i''t-Taun*, fols 85A–86A, 87A–B, 88B–90A, 91A; Al-Yahudi, *Micennetü't-Ta'un ve'l-Veba*, fols 82B–83A.
58. Mehmed Süreyyā, *Sicill-i Osmanī, İstanbul, 1308/1890–1315/1897*, vol. 1, pp. 184–5.
59. Ahmed, *Risale fi İlmi Tılsım ve Def'i''t-Taun*, fols 85A, 87A–B, 98B.
60. Ahmed, *Risale fi İlmi Tılsım ve Def'i''t-Taun*, fol. 81 B.
61. Jacques Gaffarel, *Unheard-of Curiosities: Concerning the Talismanical Sculpture of the Persians; The Horoscope of the Patriarkes; and the Reading of the Stars. Written in French, by James Gaffarel. And Englished by Edmund Chilmead, Mr. of Arts, and Chaplaine of Christ-Church Oxon*, pp. 150, 152–8.
62. T. Fahr, 'Huruf (Ilm al-)', *Encyclopedia of Islam* (online edition).

63. Gaffarel, *Unheard-of Curiosities*, pp. 153–4.
64. Ahmed, *Risale fi İlmi Tılsım ve Def'i''t-Taun*, fols 85B–86A.
65. Gaffarel, *Unheard-of Curiosities*, p. 165.
66. Mantran, *Yüzyılın İkinci Yarısında İstanbul*, pp. 233–6.
67. Mantran, *Yüzyılın İkinci Yarısında İstanbul*, p. 236.
68. Halil İnalcik, 'Bayazid II', and 'Istanbul', *Encyclopedia of Islam*.
69. Pamela H. Smith, *The Business of Alchemy: Science and Culture in the Holy Roman Empire*, pp. 5–13.
70. Kemp, *A Brief Treatise*, p. i.
71. Smith, *The Business of Alchemy*, pp. 209–17.
72. Gaffarel, *Unheard-of Curiosities*, pp. 166–7.
73. Gaffarel, *Unheard-of Curiosities*, pp. 18–20.
74. Yates, *Occult Philosophy*, pp. 37–46, 63–9, 116–19; Frances Yates, *Giordano Bruno and the Hermetic Tradition*, pp. 130–43.
75. Gadbury, *London's Deliverance*, pp. i, 24, 31; William Lilly, *England's Propheticall Merline, foretelling to all Nations of Europe untill 1663. The Actions depending upon the Influence of the Conjunction of Saturn and Jupiter, 1642/3. The Progresse and Motion of the Comet 1618. Under Whole Effects we in England, and Most Regions of Europe now suffer. What Kingdomes must yet partake of the Remainder of the Influence, viz. of War, Plague, Famine, etc. When the English Common-wealth may expect Peace, and the City of London Better Times. The Beginning, and End of the Watry Trygon: An Entrance of the Fiery Triplicity, 1603. The Nativities of some English Kings, and some Horary Question inserted: performed by William Lilly, Student in Astrologie*, p. 26.
76. Bernard Capp, *English Almanacs, 1500–1800: Astrology and the Popular Press*, pp. 23–5.
77. Lilly, *England's Propheticall Merline*, pp. 60–1.
78. Gadbury, *London's Deliverance*, pp. 12–17, 39–40.
79. Henry Oldenburg, *The Correspondence of Henry Oldenburg*, vol. 2, pp. 523, 526–7.
80. Graunt, *Natural and Political Observations*, p. 24.
81. John Gadbury, *Vox Solis: or, an Astrological Discourse of the Great Eclipse of the Sun, which happened on June 22. 1666: in 10 Deg. of the Watry Signe Cancer. Shewing what Effects may most probably attend it, and unto what Persons, Kingdoms and Countries, they are chiefly directed*, pp. 25–7.
82. Gadbury, *London's Deliverance*, pp. 25–7.
83. Christopher Barker, *England and Wales Sovereign by the Queene: A Proclamation against the Bringing in of Wines from Bordeaux in Respect to Plague being there*.
84. Yates, *Occult Philosophy*, pp. 84–5; Yates, *Giordano Bruno*, pp. 1–156, 275–90.
85. Capp, *English Almanacs*, pp. 27, 29, 41–5.
86. Gadbury, *London's Deliverance*, p. 27.
87. Dols, *The Black Death in the Middle East*, pp. 281–302.

CHAPTER

5

HAMDAN BIN EL-MERHUM OSMAN AND THE OTTOMAN QUARANTINE REFORM

INTRODUCTION

The 1838 Ottoman quarantine reform was truly a turning point in the Empire's history of epidemic disease. One might gather that Sultan Mahmud II adopted the quarantine from western European advisers and physicians; as is evident from the recommendations presented to the Ottoman ruler with regard to implementation of the institution two years earlier by the Austrian doctor Anton Lago.[1] Egyptian rival Muhammad Ali had launched his own quarantine under the guidance of foreign officials some seven years earlier. Mahmud II's predecessor Sultan Selim III had tried to do so in 1806. Many observers – Ottoman and Western – claimed that by 1840 the innovation had succeeded in eradicating plague permanently from the Empire.[2]

One seriously needs to address a number of issues in this account. Were the Ottomans and western Europeans, particularly the powerful British naval and commercial interests, unified in their support of the quarantine? One notices a number of Ottoman medical treatises in favour of this measure and a number of Anglo-American writers who were not. What exactly accounts for this discrepancy, and how did the geopolitical realities of the time, namely, the Ottoman push for reform and the concurrent British desire for commercial and colonial expansion, reflect this tension? Could one compare the Anglo-American critics' characterisation of the quarantine as a social disciplinary and ethnically divisive institution to Ottoman realities?

The following chapter will pursue these themes by discussing two interrelated sets of guiding questions. First, were Westerners or the Ottoman and other Muslim reformers primarily responsible for authoring and/or implementing quarantine and other contagionist public health policy reforms? How did such a question of control reflect upon the broader debate about nineteenth-century Ottoman reform as modernisation or Westernisation? Secondly, did quarantine and contagionist reforms lead to medical policing, where the state increasingly encroached upon civil society and individual liberty, as supposedly seen in the western European experience, or did it instead help to promote more popular participation in governmental affairs? Did such reform also promote ethnic divisions, as they were originally designed to build maritime nation-states, or could they be adopted to an alternative context, such as the multi-ethnic Ottoman Empire?

WESTERNISATION VERSUS MODERNISATION

One could easily be tempted to see the entire Muslim reform movement as an example of Westernisation, the wholesale adoption of modern European reforms, institutions and languages regardless of the socioeconomic and cultural context of the host country. Certainly, Westerners were often responsible for implementing quarantine and other contagionist institutions, such as the lazaretto and the bill of health system. It was no accident that the French armies that conquered Egypt in 1798 and Algeria in 1830 were the first to establish such measures in the Middle East. One might surmise that European diplomats and expatriate communities in the Ottoman Empire either directly introduced contagionist institutions or sent their recommendations indirectly to imperial officials, who copied them outright. Such actions could conceivably have led to a quarantine system throughout the Islamic world after 1830, which quickly eliminated plague as a result. Allegedly, Western know-how, which had conquered plague in London after 1665 and Marseilles in 1720, had finally extended beyond the continent.[3]

Yet a careful analysis of existing Ottoman sources supports the idea that Muslim reformers embraced quarantine and other modernising reforms in order to revitalise the state and to compete with their European neighbours. These modernisers adopted innovations, not simply by borrowing directly from Western ideas and institutions, but by the selective appropriation of new techniques within a local context. Ottoman, Egyptian and Tunisian reformers all pushed for quarantines and sought to have their own control. The long-term success of quarantine and other mercantilist measures was dependent on effective state formation. Quarantines were in fact mercantilist tools that protected and promoted internal economic development, and often flew in the face of free trade. Unfortunately, Ottoman dependence on Britain to ward off the Russian and Egyptian threat to imperial existence led in turn to sizable trade concessions to the British in the Balta Liman Treaty of 1838. These concessions would force the Ottomans to grant the British and other European powers partial supervision over the quarantines through the establishment of the Constantinople Superior Health Council. The European declaration of 'victory' over plague in the 1840s, and their dominance of the international sanitary conferences that followed in the ensuing decades, were reflective of this outside hegemony.[4]

Nevertheless, one needs to detail the arguments for Muslim quarantines as simply an altruistic, progressive Western idea. This is first evident in an analysis of native accounts of quarantine as an aspect of French colonisation of Egypt and Algeria, descriptions of the Europeans who introduced quarantine and lazarettos to the Ottoman Empire between 1807 and 1830, and the wholesale Ottoman adoption of the standard Western quarantine model by 1838.

Admittedly, at least two native accounts of French colonisation readily identified quarantines with Western society. Al-Jabarti, a prominent Arab notable who was an eyewitness to Napoleon's invasion of Egypt in 1798, recalled that:

> They [the French] exercise the greatest severity in the application of sanitary measures [which] harass the people and frighten them. When someone fell ill, the doctor visited him, and if he was recognised as stricken with plague, he was immediately transferred to quarantine without any of his family being able to see him afterwards . . . If he recovered, he returned home; otherwise they had him buried, fully clothed . . . His house remained closed for four days, and all his clothes were burned, . . . If any passer-by was imprudent enough to touch the door of the house or to overstep the boundaries drawn around it, he was immediately arrested by the guards and sent to quarantine. Those individuals who undertook to wash the dead, to carry them or bury them, left their quarantine only to perform their functions. These measures . . . induced many inhabitants to leave Cairo or to settle in the villages.[5]

Here Al-Jabarti describes the measures taken by the French in minute detail, but we do not get a real sense of whether he believed they were effective or not. What is most striking about this passage is instead Al-Jabarti's disillusionment with the inhumane and selfish treatment of the victims:

> As for the French it is their custom not to bury their dead but to toss them on garbage heaps like the corpses of dogs and beasts, or to throw them into the sea. Among the other things which they said is that when someone becomes sick, they must inform the French who then send an authorised representative to examine him and to find out whether he has plague or not. They then decide what to do with him.[6]

While some historians have interpreted Al-Jabarti as someone who identified quarantine as totally alien to Islamic religious sensibilities – the beliefs that the faithful should not abandon those stricken with a horrible disease and that one should not take preventive measures against plague as it was the will of God – one should also not forget Al-Jabarti's own personal motives in writing his work. Al-Jabarti, who wrote his work in part to criticise Muhammad Ali's government as a conservative critic of reform, also thoroughly discussed French bureaucratic political reform[7] – a hint that he might have actively participated in the short-lived Napoleonic government of Egypt in the wake of the 1798 invasion. Thus, it may well have been in his interest to distance himself from the most controversial aspects of the French occupation.

Hamdan Bin Osman Hoca, an Algerian who actively resisted the French shortly after they had occupied his country in 1830, had a far more positive impression:

> The measures the Europeans have implemented [in Algeria] against plague have helped them avoid plague [in Europe] for several hundred years. For example, they do not allow anyone from the countryside to enter a city unless they prove that they are not ill. The Europeans invented such quarantines in order to determine which people had the disease.[8]

Like Al-Jabarti, Hamdan credited the Europeans with the innovation: 'The quarantine first emerged in Europe and does not correspond to Islamic countries.'[9] However, he strongly believed that Muslims should also adopt the measure. Here he cited his own personal experience:

> I myself took measures to prevent plague at home in Algeria. I did not leave my household and bought items that were carried by ship [from France], and not by land. I purchased no cloth or fabrics and avoided hiring maids from the provinces . . . I would fumigate myself and not touch anyone, except when I had to go Friday prayers or funerals. Due to this, no one in my household was struck by plague.[10]

This passage shows Hamdan's own belief that the French quarantine did in fact save lives. Nonetheless, it is curious to note that the protectionist measures also included purchasing French cloth and fabrics and avoiding employing native Algerian maids. Hamdan, who wrote these passages in his own proposal for the Ottomans to implement plague, may have been aware of the mercantilist nature of this innovation. He likely saw such Western measures as a formula for ensuring a country's public health and commercial success.

Early nineteenth-century critics of quarantines in the Ottoman Empire confirmed that the quarantine and other contagionist institutions, such as the lazaretto or pest house, were indeed Western ideas. Charles Maclean, a prolific British doctor, who actively lobbied for expanding the Levant Company's trade with the Ottoman Empire in 1817, wrote that the Ottoman sultan had toyed with the idea only after a European diplomat had proposed it to him:

> Yet such was a measure seriously proposed, by the Austrian government to that of Turkey, in the reign of Selim [III (1789–1807)] with a view of extirpating epidemic diseases. That good, but in some respects weak, prince desirous of adopting every innovation, which he considered an improvement, however impractical, had himself no disinclination to entertain this proposition of the Austrian cabinet, which was formally presented to the Porte by the present worthy Internuncio Baron Stürmer.[11]

Furthermore, Maclean and James DeKay, an American who visited Istanbul in 1831–2 in the aftermath of the US trade agreement with the Ottoman Empire in May 1830 that guaranteed them most favoured nation trading status, also testified that western Europeans (also known as 'Franks') and local non-Muslims had established lazarettos of their own. Maclean complained extensively:

> Concerning these infernal depositories . . . miscalled pest hospitals in the Levant, it is proper that I should here say a few words. Their purpose is to serve as receptacles for all the miserable human beings, who are thought fit to objects of excommunication, by their families or employers, for having the misfortune to be attacked with the plague. They constitute the intermediate stage to the burying ground; to which these unfortunate victims of barbarity, are, after being almost always despoiled of their property, and often unfairly of their lives, generally in a few days duly transferred. These depots, constituting one of the most direful consequences of the doctrine of contagion, are of course only in use amongst the inhabitants of those persuasions, who entertain that pernicious belief: and their non-adoption by the Mohammedans is one of their circumstances, which contribute to except that branch of the Levant population, beyond their neighbors, from the ravages of pestilence . . . None who enter them, indeed, are ever expected to return.[12]

DeKay, like Maclean, viewed the lazaretto as a cynical plot to abandon the sick on the pretext that Western medical knowledge of the plague alone could save its victims:

> Leaving this scene, we passed under the walls of the plague hospital, built exclusively for Franks who may be affected with this disease. Over its melancholy walls we noticed the golden-berried ivy, the true ivy of the ancients, and this is the only locality about Constantinople in which I have seen it flourishing. The melancholy fate which has attended every patient admitted into this hospital gives some color to the reports which the Franks circulate of its character. According to their account, no patient has ever been known to leave this place alive, and the *voi che entrate* of Dante would seem to be the most appropriate inscription over its walls.[13]

One can confirm that certain Ottomans circles opposed quarantines and lazarettos, claiming that they were Western innovations that contradicted Muslim values. Osman Bin Süleyman Penah, the chief of Selim III's dockyards in Istanbul, the chief engineer and financial officer in charge of the Imperial Arsenal, was a most outspoken critic. Osman was personally opposed to the establishment of the Empire's first official lazaretto and medical school in the Arsenal in 1806, where Ottoman naval academy students were trained by European doctors in infectious diseases, surgery and anatomy. He in all likelihood wrote his 1804 tract against understanding plague as a contagious disease in full knowledge that the lazaretto would be established. Some three years after Osman wrote he would join Ataullah Şanizade, a former translator of Austrian medical texts, in engineering a coup against Selim III in reaction to the foreign presence and in the name of Islamic orthodoxy.[14]

Mahmud II took great care to include key Ottoman Muslim officials when he restarted contagionist reforms in the 1830s. Hamdan, recognised for his support of the Ottoman cause in Hacı Ahmed's armed struggle in western Algeria and for a condemnation of colonial rule published in French, wrote his work on plague, this time in Ottoman Turkish, to counter any opposition from conservative religious quarters. Behçed Efendi, Mahmud II's chief physician, wrote a second published work in both Ottoman Turkish and French to explain that both cholera and plague were contagious diseases. At the same time, the Empire's chief religious official, the *şeyhül-islam*, issued a *fetva* proclaiming that there was no 'harm to take refuge in God's favour from His wrath and attempt to take preventive measure when plague strikes'.[15] These actions overcame conservative Muslim opposition to the 1838 quarantine despite the fact that Lago, and apparently some Viennese physicians, were also involved. Lago's work, a forty-page treatise on how modern the institutions and rules of modern quarantine and lazarettos could be implemented in the Empire, was apparently not widely distributed beyond the bureaucratic circles directly involved in the project.[16]

Finally, it is also evident that Hamdan, one of Mahmud II's chief advocates of quarantine and other contagionist reforms, based his proposal on western European standards. The European maritime quarantine system, based in large part on Venetian customs, had three outstanding features. Hamdan detailed the first, namely, bills of health 'given to ships leaving port', at the outset of his description of the European system:

> Kings have their officials (*balyos*) all along the coast. They register every ship. Passengers have to provide sealed official papers indicating who they were, where they came from and certifying that there was no plague in their country. The officer is also in charge of describing where plague is.[17]

Hamdan followed up with an explanation of the second main feature, the European quarantine procedures:

> There are five categories of quarantine. First, are those that came from nearby countries with a good quarantine. Sick passengers should be detained until they verify what type of disease/illness they have. Second, are those that came from remote countries with a good quarantine. They should be put in quarantine in case they interacted with other ships during the journey. Third, are those that came from non-plague-infested countries without a quarantine. They should be quarantined for twenty days. Fourth, are those that came from a plague-infested country but have no plague on board. Passengers should be kept in quarantine for two months. Fifth, and finally, are ships with plague. They should be expelled without hesitation.[18]

Hamdan also spoke to the European quarantine practice of isolating and purifying goods and personal effects:

> If suspected, the passengers will go to the quarantine area but their belongings may be sunk or burnt. Passengers will be compensated accordingly. Guardsmen will be assigned to control the people under quarantine.
>
> Processed raw materials like wool and cotton will be controlled carefully and put outside during the quarantine; materials that do not pass on the dangerous air, such as olive oil, will not be put under quarantine.[19]

Finally, Hamdan described the lazaretto, the third main feature:

> Quarantine areas will be guarded on all sides; food will be provided for those who are under quarantine; private bathrooms will be provided . . . People under quarantine will have rooms. Additional space will be provided if requested.

> People under quarantine can interact with each other irrespective of the time they spent under quarantine. If people become sick, their time under quarantine will increase.[20]

Undoubtedly, the implementation of the Ottoman quarantine by 1838 – as seen in Hamdan's proposal – and Muhammad Ali's earlier 1812 regulations, were critical junctures in the history of medicine.[21] The Europeans acted quickly after the Egyptians and Ottomans established quarantines to put some under international supervision, and, in the Ottoman case, many observers declared that the epidemic threat was 'eliminated' by the mid-1840s. One could easily conclude from these developments that quarantine was a progressive Western idea that eventually trickled down to the Ottomans and other Middle Eastern Muslim states.[22]

A number of questions complicate this scenario, leading to a fundamental re-evaluation of the Ottoman and other Muslim quarantine reforms as a form of Westernisation to a view that takes native agency far more into account. First, one must question, for instance, whether the quarantine reforms were purely 'Western' in origin.

Some Western travellers critical of the reform tended to portray the widely acclaimed Ottoman belief in anti-contagionism as a universal truth. DeKay disingenuously voiced this opinion in relation to cholera in 1833 on the eve of Mahmud II's quarantine reform, which was aimed in part at this disease:

> Whether cholera be contagious is a question about which (whatever may be the fancies or the fears of ignorance) there is but one opinion among the Oriental physicians. They are unanimous in their belief of cholera being non-contagious; although partly to accommodate themselves to the vulgar prejudices and partly to inspire confidence, they direct fumigations and purifications by water.[23]

This statement is very odd given the fact that DeKay provided an accurate partial summary of a popular 1831 pamphlet on cholera by Behçed Efendi, published after the outbreak of cholera throughout the Empire that year. DeKay neglected to mention the section where Behçed directed the afflicted to take precautions:

> The first thing to do is to avoid the place where the disease occurred. Do not approach the sick people, and do not talk with them because this disease is contagious like the plague! This has been tried and proven. If the disease occurs somewhere and someone dies or is ill, it is indispensable to immediately wash the garments of the sick and even the house furniture.[24]

There is similar, although indirect, evidence of a native inclination towards contagionist thought during the decades leading up to the 1838 reform. Maclean spoke at one point in 1817 about a case involving the Grand Vizier, the most powerful official in the Empire besides the sultan:

> The present Grand Seignor is said to be one of those who entertains some apprehensions of this malady: and I have heard that, whilst I was in the hospital near the Seven Towers [in Istanbul], being struck with the death of his Hunkiar Imani, or Chaplain, he ordered the following maxim, extracted from the Hattisscherif, or collections of the sayings of Mohammed, preserved by tradition, to be brought to the recollection of the Mussulmaun people, from the principle mosques: 'The sick ought not to have communication from without, and he, who is well, ought to avoid meddling with the sick'.[25]

These sentiments for taking governmental action to prevent needless deaths were shared by Hamdan, one of the chief authors of the 1838 reform. He claimed that: 'Plague comes from putrid, fetid air which poisons light materials like cotton and wool [which people wear]. It then spreads to humans.'[26]

One then wonders what Hamdan, Behçed and the Grand Vizier based their beliefs in plague and cholera's contagious nature upon? Arguably, all three were convinced, at least in part, by direct experience with the disease. One is tempted to further speculate that they were also informed by European notions of the disease, since Western medicine was also alleged to be determined by experience, an objectivity many prior historians of medicine believe to be absent from Muslim society. Yet even if European notions of contagionism affected any of the three cases, one should not forget that Muslim thinkers and statesmen often remained receptive to 'foreign' ideas as a general rule. Hamdan prominently mentioned the platitude: 'Wisdom is the believer's guide. He should take it from wherever he finds it.' For him, this truth was just as applicable to earlier times as it was in his day. He pointed out that just as the Arabs took much of their learning from the ancient Greeks, so too did the Europeans base their experimental knowledge on prior scholars. He jokingly chastised that the Turks should follow in the Europeans footsteps, since 'One should take knowledge, even if it comes from the Arabs.'[27]

Nevertheless, Hamdan readily admitted European superiority in medicine and science because, to him, it was based upon experimental knowledge. In his eyes, the Ottomans should adopt quarantine, a practical application of this knowledge, and fundamentally rethink their approach towards learning new technology. Most controversially, Hamdan proclaimed that the Europeans' success was due to detaching natural philosophy (science and medicine) from religion.[28]

Here Hamdan had to convince a sceptical Muslim audience that adopting a secular approach was not a betrayal of the faith. Mahmud II, who apparently had not forgotten the opposition Selim III had faced from his own statesman Osman Bin Süleyman Penah, prefaced the publication of Hamdan's work with an official edict:

> A tract, now in press, will clarify the nature and conditions of the disease [plague] and combat certain prejudices from religious zealots. To ignore the sovereign in this regard is to show ungratefulness . . . Those who ignore [the tract] . . . are subject to chastisement for their misdemeanour.[29]

Hamdan clarified that the 'religious zealots' to which Mahmud II referred had a 'vain imagination'. He alleged that, according to them:

> The Europeans are infidels who have an irreligious, materialistic perspective. This fixed thinking harms the Muslim community by ignoring the source of detriment (plague) [and not adopting useful measures from Europe].[30]

Hamdan followed up this statement in an extended argument on how earlier famed Islamic thinkers reinforced his views. He pointed out, for instance, that Ghazali, the great fourteenth-century Abbassid mystic believed that: 'One should not deny philosophy because it is distinct from religion. If we deny the philosophers, we only increase their evil attitude towards Islam.'[31] Hamdan also cited Ali bin Ebu Talib, a companion of the Prophet Muhammad, as justifying the need for Muslims to keep an open mind towards acquiring new knowledge from others:

> If you know the truth, you know the people who tell the truth. Ignorance defeats humanity. If you do not know something, ask those who do. You are part of society and have a responsibility to it.[32]

Hamdan made a number of concessions in his proposal to accommodate religious sensibilities. He remarked at one point that imams should to be among the quarantine officials, since they needed 'to wash and prepare the dead'. He also mentioned that when he practised the quarantine in French-occupied Algeria, he did make sure to still attend Friday prayers and funerals. This was an acknowledgement that certain religious duties took precedence, even if it meant breaking some of the quarantine principles of personal isolation. To him, Ali's reminder of the Muslim duty to society, meaning the greater Islamic community, was a supreme virtue.[33] This was a familiar argument to Ottoman Muslim elites, the majority of whom were adherents of the liberal Hanafi school of Sunni Islam. Ottoman reformers since Ebussuud Efendi, the sixteenth-century chief religious official, appealed to the maxim that innovations were justified if they saved their people.[34]

Hamdan's tract was not the first to attempt to sway the Ottoman ruling elite on the quarantine issue. Osman's earlier work condemning the institution had aimed at the same audience that ultimately deposed Selim III. Hamdan and Mahmud II might have referred to Osman as a 'religious zealot', but the fact was that he was among the privileged 'enlightened *ulema*' Selim III had entrusted with the reform movement.[35] Thus, there was very little to distinguish Osman from Hamdan and other members of the Ottoman bureaucratic class except for the political and religious rhetoric which both of them used. Hence, terms like 'enlightened', 'zealot', 'backward' and 'dogmatic' were relative to the political struggles at the time at which they wrote.

What really counted towards both Osman's and Hamdan's success in persuading the Ottoman public was their shared sense of patriotism. Just as Osman was motivated by the large numbers of foreign doctors and other experts Selim III had employed to man his reform effort, so too Hamdan was convinced that the threat of European colonisation was very real. He illustrated this most clearly in his 1833 work, which protested to the French public how they had unfairly colonised Algeria:

> One would think that an honourable nation [like the French] would not violate its own treaties so that we could enjoy liberty and be treated justly. It would not matter if Pierre or Paul governed, the principle of the French government was not to touch our religion. Religion is a moral thing that one should not dispute with us. The French people's fraternity will unite us with them. Civilisation is based on people's rights, and we are not scared of a civilised nation. Such were the reflections [before we found out differently] . . . The Turks professed the same religion as us. We acknowledged their government, but our mores and religion were respected, our properties were not pillaged, our blood was not spilled, and our wives and children were not massacred.[36]

He also elaborated on the progressive nature of Ottoman rule: 'The Turks, "the so-called barbarians" maintained tolerance and effective rule in Algeria and elsewhere in the vicinity of Europe for three centuries.'[37]

Such statements published in French and distributed in Paris just in time for a parliamentary debate on reconsidering Algerian policy reveal that Hamdan understood, and fully participated within, a Western political context. He, indeed, was using his knowledge of French political and literary culture to combat the French in the most effective way he knew. His daring protest, written in collaboration with Ottoman Foreign Minister Mustafa Reşid (1800–58), later the key architect of the Ottoman reform movement, resulted in Hamdan's permanent expulsion from Algeria after his work hit the press. The act must have also won him substantial gratitude among the Ottoman public, a reputation that Mahmud II was no doubt cognisant of when he backed his quarantine tract. The fact that Hamdan and the other quarantine reformers met no substantial opposition from 'religious zealots' highlighted the success of this strategy.[38]

This leads one to question whether the Ottoman quarantine was really in the European interests. Great Britain, by far the strongest commercial power in the eastern Mediterranean, as in much of the Indian and Atlantic oceans, had a growing engagement with the Ottoman economy. By the early nineteenth century, British merchants were eager to increase their sales of cotton goods and woollens in return for a variety of raw material products, including raw cotton and mohair. The Treaty of Balta Liman of 1838 – which greatly reduced external and internal tariffs to British traders – was a logical precondition for flooding the Ottoman market with British textiles.

One can see the dramatic upturn in the sale of both cotton goods and woollen textiles imported into the Ottoman Empire.[39] The effect that this growth of imported cotton goods, from approximately 850,000 tons in 1838 to 3.8 million tons in 1855, and woollen textiles, from 38,000 tons to 135,000 tons, had on the Ottoman Empire was to inhibit domestic manufacturers. Urquhart described in detail his vision of this commercialisation of agriculture only some five years before the treaty:

> The manufacture of cotton is the principal indoor occupation of the greater portion of the East – of the above sixty-millions of men, with whom our future commerce will probably be carried on through the scales of the Levant – of men who are applying their labour to manufacture the cotton, and wool, and silk, that clothe them, while their fields lie uncultivated under a climate producing all of those articles which at present give the highest remuneration for labour. Throughout these vast and varied regions, these resources have lain dormant, as in the Turkish village; because hitherto the first object of necessity was not furnished to them cheap enough to induce them to forgo its manufacture, and turned their attention to cultivation. How important, then, is it to establish the fact, that our cottons are at a sufficiently low price to induce them to forgo the home manufacturer! . . . The village which was insulated before, now seeks to connect itself with the lines of communication with the principal marts; cultivation extends, wealth accumulates, instruction follows, desire for new objects increases, produce is raised, England's looms have called this prosperity into

existence . . . From the year 1827 to 1830, our exports have increased from 531,704 to 1,139,613.[40]

All this trade would have been hindered by the new quarantine regulations, which targeted cotton and wool in particular. Thus, it is no surprise that authors like Maclean and Urquhart, both lobbyists for increasing trade with the Ottoman Empire, would condemn quarantines as a hindrance to trade and public health. As Chapter 3 demonstrated, quarantines were largely mercantilist measures aimed at promoting domestic industries at the expense of the free market. Hamdan, as we have noted previously, was well aware of quarantine's effects when he stated that the French colonists in Algeria purchased only goods imported from France, and that French quarantine officials charged all ships a fee in order to cover costs.[41]

Hamdan and his Ottoman compatriots were also likely aware of what the British inflicted upon some of their key trading partners. Since the 1750s the British East India Company had been instrumental in destroying India's cotton manufacturing and forcing its cotton growers to export the goods to London to help fuel textile industrial production. This led to increased British profits, an eventual motive for establishing outright colonial rule.[42] In 1839, just one year after the Balta Liman Treaty and the Ottoman quarantine reform, Great Britain went to war with China, provoked again by the British East India Company, which forced the ruling Qing dynasty to accept their illicit trade of opium despite its devastating social effects. This contradicted the ongoing colonialist myth that the British, like the other imperialist European powers, were civilising their new subjects.

Hamdan and others like him stressed the need for reform in view of such commercial imperialism. Hamdan, in fact, argued that Mahmud II pushed for an Ottoman quarantine to strengthen the state:

> The Europeans overcame plague with their precautions and taught them to their progeny. As a result, their politics and trade developed. In contrast, Muslims wasted their people . . . When he [Sultan Mahmud II] saw that another country was doing better than his, he hurried to amend the circumstances within the realm [by adopting the quarantine].[43]

Likewise, Hamdan drew a parallel between quarantine and other key reforms, such as rearming the military:

> Previously the Muslims waged war with spears, arrows and swords, while the Europeans invented gunpowder, rifles and cannons. When the Muslims acquired

> these materials from the Europeans, nobody protested but said it was necessary to acquire them.[44]

Of course, it would be a mistake to accept uncritically Hamdan's inference here that the Ottomans lagged far behind their European rivals from the seventeenth century onwards. Recent studies have shown that Ottoman gunpowder technology kept roughly apace.[45] Hamdan's statement is also misleading if it referred to Mahmud II's reformed military. The sultan's abolition of the Janissary corps in 1826 was in fact a bloody slaughter of the capital's conservative opposition. His success in this endeavour paralleled the quarantine reform. Mahmud II, learning from the mistake Selim III made in allowing the janissaries to rally against his reform, this time cunningly plotted a coup to undermine his opposition.[46]

Nevertheless, Hamdan seemingly did imply that his reform, like earlier military reforms, would rely on foreign expertise, oddly enough from his old nemesis, the French: 'There is no harm in this, since [they] have training in the matter.'[47]

This reliance on European methods and the French language can also be seen in 1838, when Mahmud II reorganised his military's medical school. Mahmud II clarified his long-term goal to assimilate European/French medical and scientific knowledge into an Ottoman Turkish cultural context in this excerpt from his inaugural address at the school:

> I have given precedence to this school because it will be dedicated to a sacred duty – the preservation of human health . . . The instruction in medicine will be in French. You may ask why this should be in a foreign language . . . What we need is well-trained doctors for our troops and for our people, on the one hand, and to have the medical sciences incorporated into our own language and our own medical literature codified, on the other. Therefore, my purpose in having you study the French language is not to teach you French as such but that you may learn medicine – and in order to incorporate that science step-by-step into our own language. Medicine will be taught in Turkish in our land only when this has been done.[48]

It should be added that the medical school was under the direction of Abdülhak Molla, even though the majority of the staff were foreigners, largely French, Viennese and Italian.[49]

Hamdan also made it clear in his proposal that the quarantine was to remain under direct Ottoman supervision. In his opinion, it was necessary for the Sultan:

> To appoint a pious Muslim as the supervisor to implement a quarantine. That person should be mature, cognizant of the needs of the Islamic lands, and not prone to nepotism. He is charged with a duty to protect the Empire from plague. The supervisor will also convene a council regularly to implement and maintain the quarantine. They should meet every day to examine the newcomer's papers and decide how long subjects should stay in quarantine. The supervisor should have all necessary authority to carry out his mission to guard the Islamic land.[50]

Similarly, quarantine was only to be implemented in Istanbul, on both sides of the Straits, in order to better regulate international travel. As one would expect for border or customs officials, quarantine officers were expected to make an oath of loyalty to swear that they would not betray their cause.[51]

The fact that the British opposed Hamdan's proposal for direct Ottoman control over the quarantine should come as no surprise. Lord Ponsonby, the British Ambassador to the Porte at the time the proposal was formally discussed in March 1838, reflected the concerns of the British Board of Trade in a letter to Prime Minister Palmerston:

> I must not omit to speak of the expenses to which the commercial Franks and others will be subjected by the quarantine; and that will not conceal my fear that, whatever measures may be adapted, the execution of them will be so bad as to subject us with all the many-fold inconveniences of sanitary regulations, without giving us the benefits that are generally supposed be derived from them . . . I am fully impressed with the importance of this matter, and I shall be most happy to be assured of the probability of possibly extricating the plague from Constantinople. I am not assured of it – I doubt it extremely, and therefore I am adverse to these measures.[52]

The Board of Trade, acting upon such concerns of lost profit and enhanced Ottoman governmental control over international commerce, renewed its efforts for free trade. When the British drew up the Balta Liman Treaty in August 1838, they insisted that quarantine be supervised by the Constantinople Superior Health Council – a body that included representatives of all the major European powers. Mahmud II, under extreme pressure from the Russian Navy at that time, conceded to the British request.[53]

This frustrated tale of quarantine reform certainly belies the view that the western Europeans were responsible for implementing the institution in the Middle East, thereby eliminating plague by 1840. Admittedly, Hamdan and other Ottoman innovators, like Muhammad Ali in Egypt and Husayn Bey in Tunisia before him, did adopt the institution from western Europe.[54] But they, like their mercantilist predecessors, sought to use quarantine as a tool to reinforce national sovereignty rather than tear it down. As Hamdan's case illustrates, he and other reformers were willing to use Western-inspired reforms, and their knowledge of the current European political and commercial context, to resist Western influence. This is a paradox that one can see throughout world history, such as when later Russian Marxists based their own modernisation and independence from the West on an ideology born in the West.

The final British protest of the quarantine was quite hypocritical, given the fact that they had used their own quarantine as an instrument of their own protectionist commercial policy but prevented the Ottomans from using the institution to stem a flood of British cotton and woollen textiles. Their declaration that two years of a weakly enforced quarantine in Istanbul had ended the nearly 500-year reign of the Ottoman Empire as 'the seminary of plague' seems simply too convenient a fit for British trading interests.[55] One might reluctantly conclude that the disease was largely a socially constructed phenomena.

However, one must note that there was no mention in Hamdan's proposal of any domestic institution, in particular the quarantine of homes which Al-Jabarti was so horrified by when he witnessed the practice in occupied Egypt. Only Lago, the foreign doctor, recommended discriminatory practices against the poor as a risk group, but the reformists did not include his ideas.[56] The Ottomans might have allowed such practices among the European expatriates and the non-Muslim Greek, Armenian and Jewish communities, but there was little evidence of a systematic practice among the Muslims themselves.

QUARANTINES AND ILLIBERALISM

Edwin Ackerknecht's seminal 1948 essay 'Anti-Contagionism Between 1821 and 1867' argues that quarantines and contagionist thought often led to illiberalism and the police state – a thesis that infers that the 1838 Ottoman quarantine legislation may have reflected a similar tendency within the empire.[57] One of Ackerknecht's main sources was the early nineteenth-century British writer Charles Maclean, who, besides writing extensively on his own investigations in Istanbul, adhered to a classical liberal argument that free trade and laissez-faire policies were essential to good governance. Maclean and others like him were opposed to quarantines and other welfare measures in general, claiming that their restrictions hurt human liberties, led to more arbitrary government and cost precious manpower and resources.

More recent literature on nineteenth-century medicine and government has largely seconded these arguments. Postmodernists like Michel Foucault and Bruno Latour saw nineteenth-century European medical reforms as encroaching upon individual autonomy and popular participation in governmental and social affairs.[58] The doctors – and quarantine officials – were also potential liberals, members of the emerging commercial class who the state co-opted by including them in the reforms. If one sees this explanation of state-initiated reform in a non-continental European context, such as Mahmud II's efforts in the Ottoman Empire, it implies that the adoption of quarantine in 1838 would inhibit a 'progressive', 'liberal' path of state formation. Some might even view Mahmud II's and Hamdan's efforts at quarantine reform as setting the stage for autocracy, social discipline and, given the Empire's rich ethnic and religious diversity, even genocide. Ackerknecht's, Foucault's and Latour's focus on issues of policing and a crippled civil society in part reflected the impact of the Second World War and its legacy of illiberalism. Disillusionment with continental European civilisation would help to foster the neoliberal James C. Scott's claim that all state-initiated modernisation projects, regardless of geographic considerations, were doomed to failure.[59]

Yet, as Peter Baldwin has recently pointed out, such dichotomies and broad generalisations deserve extensive reconsideration.[60] One might begin by remembering that Ackerknecht's nineteenth-century British liberals often wilfully obscured the mercantilist roots of their own society. As Chapter 3 has demonstrated, England's rise as an overseas commercial power rested upon seventeenth-century mercantilist reform, such as the Navigation Acts and quarantine legislation. These reforms – and the mercantilist discourse of both contagionist and anti-contagionist thought – helped to spawn the very dichotomised, ideologically charged arguments that Maclean and other nineteenth-century liberals made about their own society and how it compared with the Ottoman Empire. These writers' categorisation of the Ottomans as an anti-contagionist 'other' led them to dismiss out of hand the Ottoman attempts at modernisation – and quarantine reform.

Admittedly, Maclean and his fellow British liberals effectively illustrated that the English Quarantine Acts had had a policing aspect since the first years of their existence. By 1603, only seven years after London had initiated the Bills of Mortality, a law was passed which forbade members of infected households from leaving their habitations for six weeks.[61] The houses were to have:

> A large red cross, and Lord have mercy upon us on the door; and watchmen attending day and night to prevent anyone's going in and out, except physicians, surgeons, apothecaries, nurses, searchers, etc. allowed by authority: and this was to continue at least a month after all the family was dead or recovered.[62]

When Richard Mead authored the Quarantine Act of 1721, which regulated Levantine cotton and wool imports, he pushed for an extension of these disciplinary powers to quarantine entire city districts:

> But the greatest care must be taken that none pass without conforming themselves to this order, both by keeping diligent watch, and by punishing with the utmost severity, any that either have done so, or attempted it. And the better to discover such. It will be requisite to oblige all who travel in any part of the country, under the same penalties, to carry with them certificates, either of their coming from places not infected, or of their passing the line by permission.[63]

This call for 'internal passports' and emergency policing powers targeted the poor in particular, since, in his opinion, they were the most vulnerable and disorderly risk group:

> All possible care ought still to be taken to remove whatever causes are found to breed and promote contagion. In order to do this, the overseers of the poor (who might be assisted herein, by other officers) should visit the dwellings of all the meaner sorts of inhabitants, and where they find them stifled up too close, and nasty, should lessen their number, by sending some into better lodgings, and should take care by all manner of provision and encouragement, to make them more cleanly and sweet . . . When the sick families are gone, all the goods of the houses, in which they were, should be burned; nay the houses themselves, if that can conveniently be done.[64]

One may speculate that Mead reflected the common concern that London was growing too quickly for its own good even in 1720 – some sixty years before the dramatic increase in working-class immigration to the city was in full force during the Industrial Revolution. Imposing new regulations might keep this growth to a more reasonable level and assure the state and the more well-to-do that order would be maintained.

Later eighteenth-century advocates of quarantine reform, such as John Howard and Dr Patrick Russell, concurred that the poor were of special concern. Howard, for instance, mentioned that 'the air about poor patients is more infectious than about the rich'.[65] He later described his reasons:

> The rich are less liable to the plague than the poor because they are more careful to avoid infection, and have larger and more airy apartments, and because they are more cleanly and live better on food, with plenty of vegetables.[66]

Russell largely agreed with Mead on the need to re-house the poor on grounds of the common good and public health:

> They perhaps might be lodged in barracks, or otherwise, in a way fully as comfortable as in their wretched dwellings in town, and, in case of a return of the plague, their being already in the country would save the police an infinite deal of trouble afterwards, as well as greatly facilitate attempts to extinguish the distemper, at its resuscitation in particular parishes. At any rate, it would be some check on the progress of contagion, the propagation of which is known to be much promoted by the intercourse of the lower class of the poor.[67]

Russell's commentary on barracks is especially important given the popularity of new British welfare legislation when he wrote his work in the 1760s. State 'drafts' of the poor into such housing, like the practice of indenturing, colonisation or impressment, were common practices in England during that time.[68]

Nevertheless, quarantine advocates like Mead and Russell understood that there were limits to policing powers during epidemics. Mead recognised, for instance, that an overly harsh policy towards the poor could alienate them:

> The methods taken by the public, on such occasions, have always had the appearance of a severe discipline, and even punishment, rather than of compassionate care . . . [They] must naturally make the infected conceal the disease as long as was possible.[69]

Mead's opponents in the House of Lords came to a similar conclusion, arguing that they should quarantine only the sick, and opposed neighbourhood quarantines or resettling the poor away from affected areas:

> Because such powers as these are utterly unknown to our constitution, and repugnant, we conceive, to the lenity of our mild and free government; a tender regard to which was shown by the act Jac. I, which took care only to confine infected persons within their own houses, and to support them under that confinement, and lodged the execution of such power solely in the civil magistrate.[70]

Despite these hesitations, quarantine opponents only took a categorical stand against policing and social discipline at the beginning of the nineteenth century. For instance, Maclean posited that even the earliest acts of isolating London's sick were inhumane and ineffective:

> In 1665, the plague, in London, spread most rapidly, and proved most fatal, the very period that the shutting up of houses, supposed to be infected, and other restrictions upon intercourse, were most rigorously enforced: and it was after the

houses were again laid open, and the people abandoned all other precautions, in despair, that the spreading of the disease, and its mortality, suddenly diminished, and ceased.[71]

Maclean also elaborated on how the eighteenth-century focus on the poor actually worsened England's social situation:

> But the effects of this dread of contagion fall with ten-fold destruction upon the poor. They are not enabled to hold out, by present, or hopes of future reward, lures to meretricious attendance; and, as dread is generally more powerful than natural affection, they are not only almost certain of being left without attendance, but even without subsistence. If only suspected, they are deprived of employment: and if they have the good fortune to recover, they are still shunned as dangerous: so that the lot of those, whom an epidemic may have spared, is often beggary or starvation.[72]

The bottom line was that government-guided attempts to deal with the 'dangerous rabble' – stigmatised as an unwanted 'risk group' – created greater dependency on welfare measures and possibly planted the seeds of revolution. One might also infer, although Maclean does not mention it *per se*, the Malthusian argument that government spending on the poor was a waste, since they would perish anyway due to inadequate food supplies.[73]

Critics and advocates of quarantine were quick to tar their opponents with the brush of patriotism: contrasting societies in the debate was a constant thread. For example, many stressed the 'foreign' bureaucratic or illiberal aspects of quarantine. One can see anti-Catholic rhetoric when Mead's anonymous opponent claimed that quarantine advocates and officials worked 'under the power of the Pope and the ecclesiastical state', and that their beliefs were 'newly broached in arbitrary states and governments'.[74] Maclean similarly concluded that the chief opponent of his liberal arguments against quarantine was the Pope.[75] Both these critics hoped to tap into the British antipathy towards Catholicism present since the Reformation. Others made the same connection to French mercantilists, who, of course, rivalled the British in the Levant trade throughout the eighteenth century. The House of Lords exposed this bias in 1721 when they criticised Mead's Quarantine Act:

> These methods were copied from France, a kingdom whose pattern, in such cases, Great Britain should not follow; the government there being conducted by arbitrary power, and supported by standing armies.[76]

DeKay slightly tailored this line of argument when he went after governments who supported quarantines throughout the Mediterranean in 1831–2:

> The rulers of Europe, who in all past times made quarantines the pretext for shutting out the contagion of liberal ideas, eagerly seized upon this disease as a reason for doubling their quarantines, and, if possible, increasing their rigor. This has been carried, during the present year, to such an extent, that all commercial intercourse was at a stand, and the short-sighted despots discovered at last that there were bounds and limits even to their arbitrary decrees.[77]

Here DeKay took aim at the rigorous controls many post-Napoleonic era European states put in place to prevent liberal opposition movements. He went on to castigate quarantine as a parasitical institution that hindered both commerce and the free flow of ideas:

> It may safely be asserted that quarantines are jobs designedly intended to give salaries to physicians, superintendents, and guards, at the expense of the unfortunate sufferers. In the Levant, in addition to these powerful pecuniary reasons, others of a political nature tend to keep up the monstrous farce. During the thirty- or forty-days quarantine, ample time is allowed to procure all the information necessary respecting the opinions and views of the prisoner. He is surrounded by spies; and the men who supply him with food at twice its value pander to the guilty fears of his government, by furnishing them with the minutest chit-chat of the stranger, which may throw any light upon his political opinions. It is, in fact, not so much the contagion of disease as of liberal opinions that is dreaded, and in this view quarantines are to be despised as the instruments of despotism.[78]

The nineteenth-century liberals saw the Ottomans in a much more positive light.

Their idealisation of the 'Turks' as laudable anti-contagionists stretched from the sultan down to the man on the street. DeKay, indeed, viewed Sultan Mahmud II as the 'one crowned head who refused to establish quarantines, and contented himself with laughing at the beards of his royal brethren'. He praised him in 1831–2 for not going 'the whole length of what is considered in Europe as the index of civilization, to wit, custom houses and quarantines'.[79] He argued that it was no surprise therefore, that:

> The Turks content themselves with sending those attacked with plague to breathe the pure air of the country, and purified their dwellings. In the meantime they permit vessels to arrive from all parts of the world, and to depart, undisturbed

> and unimpeded by the delay, the expense, the imprisonment, and the official impertinence and extortion of a quarantine establishment.[80]

Even Maclean, who generally viewed the Ottoman rulers more negatively, favourably compared their government's abstention from policing 'domestic' quarantines to the history of such measures in his own country:

> Under the Turkish dominion, however, each individual is left to act, according to his discretion, with respect to the government of himself, and of his family, in times of pestilence. He is not shut up in his house, surrounded by watchmen, shunned by his neighbours, or deserted by his children, if supposed to be infected. He may seek a more salubrious air, without the danger of perishing for want of food, or been driven back into a pestilential atmosphere by neighbouring peasants, both of which happened in the plague of London, in 1665.[81]

Such positive commentaries on the anti-contagionist Sultanate were matched by generalisations about the so-called popular Ottoman belief in anti-contagion. In DeKay's eyes, for example, the average Turk on the street did not heed constant rumours of plague:

> I see the Turk marching along with an air of the greatest nonchalance, elbowing his way through the crowd as if unacquainted with the existence of such a disease as plague, or rather to show his constitutional fortitude and his utter contempt for the puerile precautions adopted by his timid neighbors; but then, on the other hand, everyone knows that Osman is an infidel, and of course not a civilized being, consequently he has not intellect enough to comprehend when he is in danger, and when he is safe. With this sapient conclusion, the Franks of Pera, who are far from being the representatives of the collective wisdom of Europe, persist in their childish terrors, and continue their absurd precautions.[82]

DeKay's satirical defence of the so-called 'fatalist Turk' as a 'noble savage' is matched by assertions that the 'Turk', in contrast to the contagionist European, helped those in need, regardless of the danger plague posed to his or her own well-being. The 'humane Turk' did not desert his or her friends or family when they had the misfortune to be struck by the plague.[83]

One cannot take such statements at face value. DeKay, writing in 1831–2, and Maclean, writing in 1817, were very likely both aware of the Ottoman Turks impending quarantine reforms, and a number of Turks, particularly bureaucratic elites if not the average Ottoman, suspected that plague was indeed a contagious disease.[84]

This critique especially holds true for DeKay's idealisation of the Ottoman Empire as a liberal republic. Ingratiating himself to Sultan Mahmud II he claimed that:

> Like all his subjects, the Sultan is extremely temperate in eating, and his establishment is far from being on that expensive and magnificent scale which we are accustomed to attribute to Oriental courts. I have been assured by an officer of his household, that the expenses of his table rarely exceed ten piastres, or about fifty cents, a day; and from various anecdotes which I have elsewhere heard, I should not be disposed to believe that his annual expenses exceed those of the President of the United States. [85]

The modesty he mentioned of the sultan stems from Islam, a religion he believed empowered its adherents to constructively participate in political life:

> Of the influence of Islamism on the actions and lives of its professors we have already treated, and it only remains to add that its direct tendency to counteract and mitigate the severity of the despotic governments, which in East have always found a congenial soil. It produces an equalizing effect, and is in fact a sort of religious republicanism, only extending much further than in our country [the United States] where a difference of complexion is fatal. It ennobles all who profess it, and furnishes an absolute title to any office short of the throne itself.[86]

Thus, he concluded that Muslim values were key to realising social and political inequalities. His comment here that Americans, who allegedly also tapped into the 'Protestant' mantra of 'an equality of all believers', could not overcome questions of racism (that is, a 'difference of complexion'). He also highlighted the Ottoman's 'perfect toleration' of other religious faiths in this regard.[87]

Perhaps even more important is DeKay's argument that Ottoman Muslim personal practice of giving to the poor obviated the need for state intervention:

> The Turkish proverb, 'all that you give you will carry with you' beautifully expresses their belief in the importance and efficacy of alms. The giving of alms is frequently impressed as one of the highest duties of the believer; and we are told that at one time the practice was carried to such an extent as to produce a decree from the ulemah that not more than a fifth should be given to the poor. At present we are informed that is upon an average about two and a half percent. In no country in the world are beggars treated with more kindness and consideration than in Turkey, or their wants more speedily relieved. Poverty, in fact, appears to be a passport under which a beggar will not only thrust himself into the highest

> public offices, but even into the council chamber of the divan, with the certainty of having his wants relieved.[88]

This general sense of philanthropy thus explained why the Ottomans would not need or want a quarantine. They understood from the outset that the state had a sacred duty to protect the sick and poor.

The liberals, and Western commentators in general, did not spare differentiating the non-Muslim Ottoman minorities and European expatriates from the Turks. In particular, DeKay condemned the groups for their inhumane and irrational fear of plague:

> When any . . . [non-Muslim or European] is seized with it [plague], he is immediately abandoned to his fate. No medical man will dare approach him, on pain of being himself ruined; all rational mode of cure is neglected as useless, and the aid of medicine is given up in despair. That sympathy which our common nature yields to the sick is here denied. The [one] sick of the plague is put out of the pale of pity, and only looked upon as some noxious being, whom it ought be not only allowable, but meritorious, to destroy; and so the disease proceeds, rendering asunder the ties of families, extinguishing the common charities of life, eradicating the best feelings of our nature, till at length it has become one of the most dreadful moral as well as physical evils – at once the scourge and the scorn of humanity.[89]

This echoed Boccaccio's age-old criticism that the popular belief in contagionism led to the immoral abandonment of the stricken.[90] DeKay then alluded to a personal case of plague involving his own next-door neighbour, Dr Visconti, who had dutifully attended many patients in the European dominated city quarters of Istanbul. When the 'fatal bubo' appeared near his bowels, no one would dare approach until they were offered the sizeable sum of 1,000 piastres.[91]

To DeKay, the non-Muslim mania about plague was a fact of life:

> It is truly surprising that people who have been from their childhood accustomed to the presence of this disease should yet live in such continual terror. The first question asked is: 'Are there any new accidents today?' For by this polite periphrasis do the ignorant and timid European residents here designate one of the greatest scourges of humanity. I have noticed, for several days past, that people of all classes walk about the streets with smelling bottles in their hands, and with rags or bits of cotton thrust in their nostrils. To a newcomer it is laughable to witness the caution with which the Franks pick their way along the streets, carefully avoiding to tread on the least particle of woolen, cotton, or

> paper, and jumping from side to side to avoid touching even the clothes of the passers-by.[92]

One should remember that there is no evidence in this or any other statement by Western travellers that the Levantine community ever was able to impose domestic quarantines by force. There are occasional hints by DeKay and Maclean that the 'municipal authorities', namely, the Greek Patriarch and the European consuls, called for quarantines, but the police were Ottoman Muslims who remained aloof.[93]

The writers also compare plague death rates among the communities. For instance, John Howard claimed that 'the Jews in Constantinople and Smyrna lose only one third . . . the Turks lose two-thirds; other nations a little more or less'.[94] DeKay and Maclean came to similar conclusions about the higher rate for Turks and for Ottoman non-Muslims and Europeans.

The authors had a number of reasons for this difference. Howard pointed out that diet largely explained the discrepancy. The Turks had very meagre eating habits followed by the Ottoman Greeks and Jews:

> The poorer sort of Greeks and Jews use much oil with their food; and this I reckon [is] a disadvantage to them. I have heard of instances of servants in European families, who through imprudence and carelessness, had been attacked with the plague, while the rest of the family have escaped it.[95]

DeKay also agreed that the plague rarely struck the 'well-fed part of the population'.[96]

However, DeKay also saw alcohol use as a major factor:

> I was cautioned against dieting myself to ward off this disease, and indeed the use of spirits was warmly recommended. It is supposed that the rigid temperance of the Turks renders them more obnoxious to its attacks; but whether that be the case or not, it is certain that the Franks, who lived upon the fat of the land, and wash it down with copious draughts of wine, are rarely affected by this disease.[97]

DeKay characterised the Greeks as the most prolific drinkers. He noted that during his neighbour's funeral that the casket bearers, 'three Greeks, [took] the precautionary measure of getting most conspicuously drunk'.[98]

This was not the only instance where the writers connected drug use to a different religious, ethnic or 'racial' group. The most popular drug use to disparage was opium, of course. Howard and Maclean alleged opium use to attack Turkish statesmen and physicians who disagreed with their arguments. On the one hand,

Howard, who pushed the Ottomans to hire Western European doctors, claimed that their Turkish counterparts were dangerously incompetent:

> The Turks have few hospitals at Constantinople. Those for the sick are a fort of caravansaries, in one of which, I saw many sick and dying objects lying on dirty mats on the floors. The surgeon seemed to be either extremely stupid, or intoxicated with opium.[99]

On the other hand, Maclean cursed the Ottoman government officials after they refused to hire him to conduct a study on plague:

> It not only appears not to have been in the policy of the Ottoman Porte, to enter into my views of increasing the population of their territory; but, sensible of the opium, which could [also] not fail to attend the rejection of my propositions.[100]

DeKay, who was still hopeful of gaining Ottoman support for his own cause, tried to address this derision with his own anti-Semitic diatribe against the Ottoman Jewish minority:

> It was here too that we saw for the first time an opium-eater. He was a miserable-looking Jew, pale and emaciated, and, although his eyes were rolling about every part of the room, he appeared to be unconscious of the presence of anyone around him. The idea of a Turk and an opium-eater is so naturally associated in our minds, that for a long period after our arrival here we were in daily expectation of meeting some Turk in the streets, maddened with opium, and ready to plunge with his yataghan into the body of the first Christian that crossed his path. It was not until after a residence of several months that we were enabled to put a just value upon the representation of those who deal in exaggeration, in order to make an impressive picture. As none fell in our way, we determined to ferret them out in their secret haunts, and even to experiment ourselves with this pleasing poison.
>
> Opium is known to be one of the staple products of Turkey; and hence, it has been logically inferred, that everybody in the country must use it habitually. The Turks, by the same ingenious process of reasoning, conclude that the Americans are the most intolerable opium-eaters in the world, because they are the greatest purchasers of that commodity.[101]

DeKay expounded his anti-Semitism in another passage about the Ottoman Jews as a 'degraded race . . . distinguished by its dirt and filth'. Oddly enough, DeKay also did not hesitate to use his fellow Americans as a foil for his idealisation of the Ottoman Turks. One may speculate that he was referring in part to his 'own' minority, the African-Americans. At one point in his text, he referred to two 'Blacks' who were the only ones to die from cholera during an outbreak in an American sloop-of-war sitting off Istanbul's Golden Horn. He explained they died because they refused to take modern medicine.[102]

The most striking aspect of the above liberal discourse on quarantines and social discipline is its superficial comparisons of the Anglo-American world to the foreign 'other'. While the writers described the 'domestic quarantine' in England, they did not refer at all to what policing measures were taken in 'despotic', 'contagionist' France and other continental European countries whose quarantines hurt their commerce. Similarly, the writers uniformly labelled the Ottomans as strictly 'anti-contagionist' during the reigns of Selim III and Mahmud II when quarantine reform was in the air. This mistake parallels misleading generalisations that Western observers made elsewhere, such as the claim that plague was endemic to the Middle East alone.

This illustrates the weakness of Ackerknecht's sources for the Ottoman Empire. Writers like Maclean and DeKay were committed first and foremost to an agenda of liberal free trade, and were more than willing to play with the facts accordingly. One could see this, for instance, in Maclean's vignette of the opium-smoking Turkish officials, and DeKay's glorification of Mahmud II and the chief court physician Behçed Efendi as strict anti-contagionists even when they knew the contrary was true. The truth according to these sources was relative – as the limited Ottoman sources we have on the subject point in an entirely different direction.

The question as to whether there were social consequences to the quarantine reforms is open to debate. Ottoman officials very occasionally mentioned poor migrants from the countryside as a potential cause of the plague. As early as 1792, an Ottoman imperial decree ordered that beggars in Istanbul who were sick with contagious diseases should be put into hospitals, while the able-bodied 'should be deported to their place of birth'.[103] Such notions lingered even after Selim III was deposed by his so-called conservative opponents. An 1812 edict complained about recent poor migrants to Istanbul who spread plague by soliciting prostitutes: 'God's wrath has punished this behaviour by striking down the population with plague for the past three to five months. Get rid of the villainous households and the disease will stop . . .'[104] Hamdan chided the religious and sexual overtones, but accepted urban immigration as a cause when plague struck colonised Algeria:

> The French hired [Algerian] maids to do shopping but would spread disease to their masters and sons after mixing with the local population in coffee houses, bath houses etc.[105]

Anton Lago also took up this issue in his treatise when he argued that the Ottomans should regard the poor as a risk group: quarantine officials should pay attention to the poor and the filthy environment in which they lived. He even recommended that the poor be isolated from those of better social standing when they were in the quarantines or lazarettos.[106]

The Ottomans were reluctant to embrace such principles within their reform efforts, however. Neither Hamdan nor any of the prominent Muslim quarantine officials seem to have promulgated discriminatory practices against the poor from 1838 until 1894, when the Europeans pushed the issue with regard to allegedly impoverished Muslim pilgrims from their colonial possessions who were seeking to visit Ottoman Mecca and Medina in order to perform their religious duties. Hamdan might have had his prejudices, but he and the other reformers were very aware that the Ottoman religious authorities – the traditional overseers of the urban poor – might be very leery of sanitary policing practices that would undermine their authority.

In contrast, it was the Europeans who stressed the so-called social and ethnic aspects of the Ottoman quarantine. Lord Ponsonby, the British Ambassador to Istanbul who derailed the 1838 quarantine, protested Sultan Mahmud II's alleged consideration of a domestic quarantine:

> The other proposal is to empower the health officials to enter any house in which they may believe the plague to have broken out and to take such measures as they may judge expedient, being authorised to act by some member of the Board of Health. This power will occasion a serious inroad upon one great and precious principle and right created by our capitulations, that is the inviolability of the domicile of the Frank; and it will probably occasion robbery, perhaps murders, and certainly infinite distress and misery to the sick.[107]

This statement strikes a familiar chord: the Ottomans, like other quarantinists, were arbitrary, despotic and could not be trusted with control. The 'Franks', namely, European expatriates and Istanbul's and Smyrna's Greek minority, were able to run hospitals of their own. There were occasional contests between the hospital authorities, who wished to extend their own influence to nearby Muslim residents, and the central authorities, who occasionally sent guardsmen to extract fees for new construction and collecting taxes.[108] Thus, it was the Europeans, and not the Ottomans, who insisted that a domestic quarantine would define the superiority of one religious community over another.

In a similar vein, I have not been able to locate any case of anti-Semitism in the source material except for Hamdan's protest to the French for occupying Algeria. His derogatory comments about Algeria's Jews as 'money grubbing' and 'exploitative' can be traced to the French use of ethnic politics to consolidate its rule.[109] One sees here a foretaste of twentieth-century Palestinian anti-Semitism, which was based on a similar resentment of outside intervention.

Liberal writers, like Maclean and DeKay, themselves contributed to the cause of Western imperialist expansion in the Middle East by highlighting ethnic, religious and class differences within the Empire. Their success in convincing their English-speaking readers to support overseas commercial efforts helped to bring greater instability. The breakdown of the Ottoman protectionist measures, and Grand Vizier Mustafa Reşid Pasha's declaration of the equality of all Ottomans, regardless of religious creed, encouraged both Christian minority separatist movements (that is, Greeks, Armenians, Marionites) and their European sponsors to take advantage of imperial weakness.[110] This sense of vulnerability, very similar to what Hamdan felt about the French occupation of Algeria, would be the true harbinger of ethnic nationalism in the century to come. In sum, it was the imperialist powers, and not the Ottoman drive towards modernisation and quarantine reform, that promoted illiberal notions of identity and governance.

CONCLUSION

The 1838 Ottoman quarantine lends important new insights into the Empire's reform movement. Native reformers like Sultan Mahmud II and Hamdan initiated the measure to strengthen the Ottoman state and to resist British commercial expansion rather than pave the way for it. Here paradoxically the Ottoman reformists followed the same path trodden by the English some two centuries earlier. The quarantine and contagionist reforms, like modernisation as a whole, may have strived to order society and increase the financial reach of the state. However, they were not bound to stress ethnic and religious differences through policing measures with the teleological aim of separatist nationalism. It was, ironically, the early nineteenth-century Anglo-American treatise writers who spoke of human and economic liberty who were the ones to encourage ethnic, religious and even racial division instead of a reinvigorated, sovereign and self-sufficient Ottoman government. Equally ironically, the Ottoman reformers who succeeded in convincing their domestic critics of the need to resist outside powers caved in to British pressure to establish the Constantinople Superior Health Council. If one could have asked Hamdan after 1840 if he agreed that the plague was gone, he might have quipped that the only 'sick' patient was the Ottoman state itself.

NOTES

1. Lago, *Risale-i Karantina.*
2. Berkes, *Development of Secularism in Turkey*, p. 121; Panzac, *La Peste dans l'Empire Ottoman*, pp. 475–83.
3. Kuhnke, *Lives at Risk*, pp. 3–4, 9–10; Panzac, *La Peste dans l'Empire Ottoman*, pp. 11–16.
4. Kuhnke, *Lives at Risk*, pp. 89–98; Panzac, *La Peste dans l'Empire Ottoman*, pp. 480–3.
5. Kuhnke, *Lives at Risk*, p. 76.
6. Abd al-Rahmān Jabarti, *Napoleon in Egypt: Al-Jabartī's Chronicle of the French Occupation, 1798*, p. 71.
7. Jabarti, *Napoleon in Egypt*, p. 14.
8. Hamdan, *Tercüme-i İthaf*, fol. 39B.
9. Hamdan, *Tercüme-i İthaf*, fol. 46A.
10. Hamdan, *Tercüme-i İthaf*, fols 56B–57A, 64B–65A.
11. Maclean, *Results of an Investigation*, p. 457.
12. Maclean, *Results of an Investigation*, pp. 47–8.
13. DeKay, *Sketches of Turkey in 1831 and 1832*, p. 162.
14. Stanford J. Shaw, *Between Old and New: The Ottoman Empire under Sultan Selim III, 1789–1807*, pp. 92, 100, 103–4, 375.
15. Uludağ, 'Son Kapitülasyonlardan biri Karantina', p. 448.
16. Lago, *Risale-i Karantina*, fols 1A, 2B, 21B–22A.
17. Hamdan, *Tercüme-i İthaf*, fol. 62A.
18. Hamdan, *Tercüme-i İthaf*, fol. 62B.
19. Hamdan, *Tercüme-i İthaf*, fols 62B, 63A–B.
20. Hamdan, *Tercüme-i İthaf*, fols 63A–64A.
21. Lago also had a similar description of the quarantine and those people and goods who should be inspected by its officials. Lago, *Risale-i Karantina*, fols 2A–19A.
22. Panzac, *La Peste dans l'Empire Ottoman*, pp. 515–18; Kuhnke, *Lives at Risk*, pp. 92–9.
23. DeKay, *Sketches of Turkey in 1831 and 1832*, pp. 336–7.
24. Panzac, *La Peste dans l'Empire Ottoman*, p. 580.
25. Maclean, *Results of an Investigation*, pp. 427–8.
26. Hamdan, *Tercüme-i İthaf*, fol. 59A.
27. Hamdan, *Tercüme-i İthaf*, fol. 43B.
28. Hamdan, *Tercüme-i İthaf*, fols 43B–46A, 59A.
29. Panzac, *La Peste dans l'Empire Ottoman*, pp. 583–5.
30. Hamdan, *Tercüme-i İthaf*, fol. 39B.
31. Hamdan, *Tercüme-i İthaf*, fol. 44B.
32. Hamdan, *Tercüme-i İthaf*, fol. 45A.
33. Hamdan, *Tercüme-i İthaf*, fols 45A, 65B.
34. İnalcik, 'The Tanzimat and its social effects', p. 12.
35. Panzac, *La Peste dans l'Empire Ottoman*, pp. 583–5.
36. Hamdan Khodja, *Le Miroir: Aperçu Historique et Statistique sur la Régence d'Alger*, p. 174.
37. Hamdan Khodja, *Le Miroir*, p. 87.
38. Panzac, *La Peste dans l'Empire Ottoman*, pp. 493–514; Abdeljelil Temimi, *Le Beylik de Constantine et Ḥadj Aḥmed Bey (1830–1837)*, pp. 7–10.

39. Frank Edgar Bailey, *British Policy and the Turkish Reform Movement: A Study in Anglo-Turkish Relations, 1826–1853*, pp. 86–7, 93.
40. Urquhart, *Turkey and its Resources: Its Municipal Organization and Free Trade; the State and Prospects of English Commerce in the East, the New Administration of Greece, its Revenue and National Possessions*, pp. 143–4.
41. Hamdan, *Tercüme-i İthaf*, fols 64B–65A.
42. Irfan Habib, 'Colonization of the Indian economy, 1757–1900', pp. 23–30.
43. Hamdan, *Tercüme-i İthaf*, fols 34B, 36B.
44. Hamdan, *Tercüme-i İthaf*, fol. 67A.
45. Rhoads Murphey, *Ottoman Warfare, 1500–1700*, pp. 13–14.
46. Berkes, *Development of Secularism in Turkey*, pp. 90–7.
47. Hamdan, *Tercüme-i İthaf*, fol. 67A.
48. Berkes, *Development of Secularism in Turkey*, p. 113.
49. Clot-Bey, the French expatriate who Mohammed Ali directed to found the first modern medical school in Egypt in 1827 came to a similar conclusion: 'In order to be lasting, useful institutions [like the medical school] should be national and independent of the cooperation of foreigners.' Kuhnke, *Lives at Risk*, p. 34.
50. Hamdan, *Tercüme-i İthaf*, fol. 65A.
51. Hamdan, *Tercüme-i İthaf*, fols 66B–67A.
52. Panzac, *La Peste dans l'Empire Ottoman*, pp. 481–2.
53. The French also made a similar protest to the Tunisian government in 1828, on the eve of its invasion of Algeria. Husayn Bey, the Bey of Tunis, replied to de Lesseps, the Consul General of France to Tunis: 'Your request was to remove the quarantine from merchant ships coming from your Mediterranean ports. We have considered your request and the answer is that we ordered the ten days to protect the people. God Almighty gave us the duty to take care of their welfare and to protect them from contagious diseases. It came to us from many authoritative sources that plague, yellow fever and other diseases are spreading. Yellow fever is severe in Gibraltar and elsewhere. We know that merchant ships have contact with other ships at sea and in port so we ordered these ten days to protect the land and the people . . . We put this order on all types of ships coming to our country. Orders cannot be done for some and not for others. If we accept your request, others would demand it and enforcing the order would become very difficult. The result would be corruption coming to our country . . . France with its ancient friendship with us, understands that we did not order the quarantine to hinder commerce. We made the order not knowing if it will work, but it might, so it's not possible for us not to do it . . .' Gallagher, *Medicine and Power in Tunisia*, p. 106.
54. Kuhnke, *Lives at Risk*, pp. 2–15; Gallagher, *Medicine and Power in Tunisia*, p. 32.
55. Mead, *Short Discourse*, p. 13.
56. Lago, *Risale-i Karantina*, fols 7A, 12B–13B, 21B–22A.
57. Erwin Ackerknecht, 'Anticontagionism between 1821 and 1867', pp. 562–93.
58. Michel Foucault, *Kliniğin Doğuşu*, pp. 7–18; Bruno Latour, *The Pasteurization of France*, pp. 3–12.
59. James C. Scott, *Seeing like a State: How Certain Schemes to Improve the Human Condition Have Failed*, pp. 1–8.
60. Baldwin, *Contagion and the State in Europe, 1830–1930*, pp. 24–5.
61. Patrick Russell, *A Treatise of the Plague*, p. 480.
62. Mead, *Short Discourse*, p. 15.

63. Mead, *Short Discourse*, p. 24.
64. Mead, *Short Discourse*, pp. 18–19.
65. Howard, *Account of the Principal Lazarettos in Europe*, p. 34.
66. Howard, *Account of the Principal Lazarettos in Europe*, p. 25.
67. Patrick Russell, *A Treatise of the Plague*, p. 551.
68. Roy Porter, *British Enlightenment*, pp. 358–9.
69. Mead, Short Discourse, p. 15.
70. Patrick Russell, *A Treatise of the Plague*, p. 501.
71. Maclean, *Results of an Investigation*, p. 456.
72. Maclean, *Results of an Investigation*, p. 429.
73. Roy Porter, *British Enlightenment*, pp. 470–5.
74. Explainer, *Distinct Notions of the Plague*, p. 126.
75. Maclean, *Results of an Investigation*, pp. 2, 107.
76. Patrick Russell, *A Treatise of the Plague*, p. 501.
77. DeKay, *Sketches of Turkey in 1831 and 1832*, pp. 337–8.
78. DeKay, *Sketches of Turkey in 1831 and 1832*, p. 340.
79. DeKay, *Sketches of Turkey in 1831 and 1832*, p. 338.
80. DeKay, *Sketches of Turkey in 1831 and 1832*, p. 339.
81. Maclean, *Results of an Investigation*, pp. 425–6.
82. DeKay, *Sketches of Turkey in 1831 and 1832*, p. 131.
83. Maclean, *Results of an Investigation*, p. 425.
84. This inference is based on DeKay's detailed summary and translation of Behçed Efendi, who was part of the 1830–1 commission studying the effectiveness of quarantines for fighting cholera and plague, and Maclean's claim about the 'contagionist' Grand Vizier. DeKay, *Sketches of Turkey in 1831 and 1832*, p. 336; Maclean, *Results of an Investigation*, pp. 427–8.
85. DeKay, *Sketches of Turkey in 1831 and 1832*, p. 155.
86. DeKay, *Sketches of Turkey in 1831 and 1832*, p. 362.
87. DeKay, *Sketches of Turkey in 1831 and 1832*, p. 362.
88. DeKay, *Sketches of Turkey in 1831 and 1832*, p. 358.
89. DeKay, *Sketches of Turkey in 1831 and 1832*, p. 175.
90. Boccaccio, *The Decameron*, pp. 6–14.
91. DeKay, *Sketches of Turkey in 1831 and 1832*. p. 189.
92. DeKay, *Sketches of Turkey in 1831 and 1832*, pp. 130–1.
93. DeKay, *Sketches of Turkey in 1831 and 1832*, pp. 130–1; Maclean, *Results of an Investigation*, p. 425.
94. Howard, *Account of the Principal Lazarettos in Europe*, p. 40.
95. Howard, *Account of the Principal Lazarettos in Europe*, p. 25.
96. Howard, *Account of the Principal Lazarettos in Europe*, pp. 175–6.
97. Howard, *Account of the Principal Lazarettos in Europe*, pp. 175–6.
98. Howard, *Account of the Principal Lazarettos in Europe*, pp. 190–1.
99. Howard, *Account of the Principal Lazarettos in Europe*, p. 64.
100. Maclean, *Results of an Investigation*, p. 44.
101. DeKay, *Sketches of Turkey in 1831 and 1832*, p. 344.
102. DeKay, *Sketches of Turkey in 1831 and 1832*, p. 332.
103. Nadir Özbek, 'The Politics of Welfare: Philanthropy, Voluntarism and Legitimacy in the Ottoman Empire, 1876–1914', p. 36.

104. Uludağ, 'Son Kapitülasyonlardan biri Karantina', pp. 445–6.
105. Hamdan, *Tercüme-i İthaf*, fol. 64B.
106. Lago, *Risale-i Karantina*, fol. 13B.
107. Panzac, *La Peste dans l'Empire Ottoman*, pp. 481–2.
108. Uludağ, 'Osmanlı Tıp Tarihinde Reaya Hastaneleri ve İmtiyazları', pp. 279–81.
109. Hamdan Khodja, *Miroir*, p. 138.
110. İnalcik, *Ottoman Empire*, p. 156.

CHAPTER

6

PLAGUE AND QUARANTINES IN THE COLONIAL ERA

INTRODUCTION

Hamdan's belief that the internationalisation of the Ottoman quarantine in 1838 signalled capitulation to the British was ill-founded. From its inception, various interests clashed at the Constantinople Superior Health Council. Austrian physicians may have run the Constantinople Superior Health Council for a short time, but it was soon headed once again by an Ottoman president, whose administrative staff were often in conflict with the foreign members of the Council.[1]

Muhammad Ali (1769–1849), who started a process of modernising reform in Egypt in a bid to take over the empire itself, established a separate quarantine in Alexandria and other public health institutions in order to combat plague, cholera and other epidemic diseases. Like the Ottomans, Muhammad Ali gave in to European pressure and allowed international representatives to help run the Alexandria quarantine. The Europeans frequently lauded Muhammad Ali for his efforts; often claiming that Muhammad Ali's French appointees to supervise the quarantine, such as Antoine Clot (1793–1868) and Louis Aubert-Roche (1818–74), were much more successful than the Ottomans in preventing the outbreak of disease.

European criticism that the newly established Ottoman public health authorities needlessly inhibited trade and the free flow of overseas traffic by imposing a ten- to fifteen-day quarantine on all traffic passing through the Straits motivated Clot (also known as Clot-Bey) and Aubert-Roche to complete a new study of the plague in Egypt in 1846. They found that Egypt's most recent plague outbreaks could be explained by environmental factors rather than contagious ones. In their opinion, the muddy banks of the Nile and the unsanitary living conditions of its inhabitants caused periodic outbreaks of the disease. Improving water supply, hygiene and building codes could prevent disease, not isolating patients and their families, or quarantining suspected boats. Soon, this new infectionist perspective would dominate public health discourse, particularly the International Sanitary Conferences, held first in Paris in 1851.

The Ottomans were reluctant to give up contagionist notions of epidemic disease, and wished to maintain their quarantine of foreign ships and even cities. They sought to tax naval traffic and even merchandise. This led to international protests – mainly from the British. British intervention was decisive during the Crimean War in protecting the Ottomans from Russian encroachment. But Ottoman protectionist measures arguably soured relations with London's commercial interests, particularly those involved with cotton exports – still central to the British textile industry. This led in part to British plans to develop cotton as a cash crop along the Nile, and, eventually to support the Suez Canal, as it was outside of Ottoman control. Such developments led in turn to the colonisation of Egypt. The Ottomans may have relaxed trade restrictions later, but they were also forced to acknowledge the loss of Egypt and the Suez Canal. In addition, the Europeans accused the Ottomans of neglecting the annual pilgrimage after cholera spread from Mecca to Europe in 1865. These issues culminated in the 1894 and 1897 International Sanitary Conferences, which finalised quarantines in the Suez and on the Red Sea coasts; developments that forced the Ottomans to revise their understanding of plague and the institutions necessary to prevent it.

The following chapter will explore the contours of this debate between Ottoman contagionists and British and French infectionists from 1838 to the 1890s about the definition and nature of plague, where the disease was endemic, who would control the Council, and how preventative measures like the quarantine could be implemented along the major sea lanes and the pilgrimage routes.

CONTAGIONISM VERSUS INFECTIONISM

Official British and French support for Clot-Bey's and Aubert-Roche's revised understanding of plague as infectious dated back to protests of the Ottoman quarantine in 1838. Lord Posonsby, the British Ambassador to the Sublime Porte, complained to the Prime Minister:

> With reference to the proposed [Ottoman quarantine] regulations, I have to instruct your Excellency to endeavour strongly to impress upon the Turkish government that they would more effectually prevent the breaking out and spreading

of the plague by introducing cleanliness and ventilation in the city and suburbs of Constantinople, than by any such violent interference as is proposed with the domestic arrangements of families. It is quite certain that the plague is much aggravated, if not actually generated, by the wants of cleanliness in the streets, by the want of sufficient ventilation in houses, and by the want of proper drainage in places contiguous to habitation; and, if the Turkish government would, in the first instance, apply vigorous measures to correct these evils, they would strike at once at the causes of the disease; whereas the measures, which they have now in contemplation, will only be productive of inconvenience and suffering to numerous individuals.[2]

The French suggested that the best way to counter the Ottomans was to help to promote 'the formation of a general congress of delegates [from] the various European states having ports in the Mediterranean, for the purpose of agreeing on some uniform system of quarantine regulations to be adopted by all'.[3] Soon there were statements by British officials based in Malta, Syria, Erzurum and Bursa lending support for a general congress that complained of the Ottoman contagionist understanding of the disease. Mr Robert, a supervisor of British hospitals in Syria, commented:

> [In regards to this frightful disease], I beg to state that the results of all my experience leads me to believe that the disease originates in local causes, and that it is endemic in Syria and Egypt; that it is not of a highly contagious nature; and that, if ever so at all, some other concurrent circumstances are necessary to render itself. Extreme and exclusive [Ottoman] opinions on the doctrine of contagion are hardly warranted by this present state of our knowledge.[4]

Lord Aberdeen, the chief official of the British quarantine, tried in 1843 to convene the first International Sanitary Conference on the subject, and readily gained French support for his proposal. However, the Austrians viewed the conference as premature until competent medical men determined both the standard duration of a quarantine for people and goods and the best way to disinfect objects 'susceptible to contagion'.[5] As a result of this concern, the French Royal Academy of Medicine appointed Clot-Bey and Aubert-Roche to answer 'all the very questions connected with the plague and with quarantines'.[6]

Clot-Bey's and Aubert-Roche's findings, based on personal observation and lengthy interviews with medical personnel and patients in Egypt from 1831 until 1846, generally endorsed the infectionist position. In their opinion, the pestiferous atmosphere of Lower Egypt was caused by the extreme 'destitution, filth and misery' of the poor 'inhabitants of the Delta':

> Their wretched hovels are so horribly disgusting as almost to defy description; they are not only surrounded by, but are actually receptacles of heaps of ordure and putrid matters. Not infrequently are the dead buried immediately under the mud floors of these dwellings of the living; and many of the graves in the cemeteries (which are always within the villages), being left open, are continually exhaling a stench that is utterly intolerable to any stranger. Then, again, the food of the Fellah is always of the worst description, and often too of the most scanty supply. Rotten cheese, decayed vegetables, semi-putrid flesh or fish; such are the articles that he lives upon. The very water that he drinks is filthy and impure. And then think of his mental and moral condition; the brutish degradation of all his faculties and affections, his hopeless servitude, his blank unmitigated wretchedness.[7]

To them, the urban centres of Lower Egypt were also in peril:

> Cairo, with its 200,000 inhabitants, is a very hot bed of the most disgusting and pestiferous impurities. From the canal, which traverses it, there is constantly streaming forth a cloud of intolerable offence; and yet this is the supply of water for the use of its people! There are no fewer than thirty-five cemeteries, of which twenty-five are within its walls. In the Coptic quarter of the town, the dead are buried under the floors of the houses; and nothing but a few boards separate the living from the putrid bodies of the deceased. From eighty to ninety corpses have been known to be huddled together in these horrible sub-domal receptacles. Can we therefore wonder that Cairo should be a generating focus of the pestilential disease?[8]

Geographical factors were also important to Clot-Bey and Aubert-Roche. They claimed that the plague never occurred above the first cataract of the Nile, which was less densely inhabited, less humid and had more flowing water and better soil. The answer, therefore, was to improve living conditions for those living in Lower Egypt by implementing modern building codes, sewage systems, and regulating food, water supply and burial of the dead. The French authorities posited that they had already done this in Algeria, where the 'present administration' had abolished quarantine and instead rebuilt towns and villages on the slopes of the hills to make sure that they were spacious enough not to be 'overpeopled'. Gavin Milroy, a prominent British critic of the quarantine system, believed that Algeria 'may become as seldom the theatre of the pestilence as almost any of the countries of Europe'.[9]

Thus, the French and British could use sanitation measures to justify a colonial agenda for Egypt. Neither the French nor the British were willing to admit that the 'natives' themselves were capable of the implementing hygienic reform necessary to free their societies of plague or other life-threatening epidemic diseases.

Moreover, Clot-Bey led an experiment by a team of European doctors to test whether or not the blood of plague patients could infect other human beings in 1835. The subjects of the experiment were five criminals who had earlier been condemned to death. Each of the five was injected with the blood of a plague patient. Only one of the five was affected. He came down with a mild case of plague three days after the injection. Clot-Bey argued that the single mild case of plague could be explained by the patient's exposure not only to the 'epidemic atmospheric influences then existing in Cairo', but also the fact that he had lived in a plague hospital – 'a focus of pestilential infection' – three days before the experiment. Clot-Bey's beliefs were confirmed when he had injected himself six times with the blood of a plague patient without any ill effects. He followed this up with an injection of puss from a bubo and this resulted in 'a slight indisposition, which he attributed to the absorption of the purulent matter, which bore no resemblance to the symptoms of plague'.[10]

Clot-Bey and the European doctors were obviously willing to dehumanise patients in order to biologically define the disease. The doctors, armed with the knowledge of modern medicine, were allowed to experiment on marginalised others – in this case non-European criminals – in order to disprove the theory that plague was contagious through human blood. Their findings were then disseminated by medical doctors like Milroy who shared the same privileges and convictions. One could also extrapolate that other marginal populations – poor or non-European colonials – could be subjected to such measures in the future. The moral right to choose whether or not to be a subject was only limited to Clot-Bey himself, his colleagues and possibly other Europeans of good social standing.

Clot-Bey and Aubert-Roche also did not hesitate to use ethnic categories to measure the impact of the plague. They drew up a table of mortality rates during the plague outbreak in Alexandria in 1835. They concluded that 14 per cent of the city's Greek population died in the outbreak, as well as 12 per cent of the Jews, Armenians and Copts, 11 per cent of the Turks, 7 per cent of the Italians and other southern Europeans, and 5 per cent of the French, British, Russians and Germans. They contrasted this sharply with those who died, including 84 per cent of the city's blacks, 61 per cent of the Malays and 55 per cent of non-elite Arabs. The great difference in mortality rates, they claimed, was based on the assumption that 'the attacks of the pestilence among all classes of the population, native or stranger, is almost uniformly observed to be inversely proportionate to their cleanliness, good living and general comfort'.[11]

This ethnic interpretation of disease often led to denials that Europe could once again be infected with plague. Milroy exemplified this trend in 1846 when he asked:

> Is there reason to believe that the plague, when imported from the east into any European port, may be communicated to a sufficiently large number of persons to give rise to a pestilential epidemic? The medical men of Egypt answer this query in the negative. Their opinion is based on the often observed fact that, when plague patients are transported to places not subject to the pestilential constitution, they die or recover without transmitting their disease to anyone. If the infected, as we have seen, cannot communicate the disease to the inhabitants of certain places in Upper Egypt, how can we believe that, when transported from Egypt to France, it will possess a power of transmission so strong as to occasion an epidemic?[12]

Thus, Milroy inferred from Clot-Bey's and Aubert-Roche's report that 'vessels arriving from infected ports' carrying plague patients should be allowed to disembark 'at any place not subject to the epidemic pestilential influence'. Milroy ridiculed those who argued that European ports should retain quarantine procedures out of undue caution.[13]

Other British writers came to similar conclusions. Netten Radcliffe (1826–84), a contemporary of Milroy, posited in 1843 that it would be 'almost impossible for plague to get a serious hold upon' Britain, given its outstanding sanitary condition. Those extremely rare cases that were imported should be regarded as mere 'pathological curiosities'. An anonymous British writer attributed this success to a 1848 public health law that enabled his government's 'sanitary authorities' to limit overcrowding, ensure adequate ventilation, and remove 'putrescent animal and vegetable matters' from homes, buildings and streets.[14]

The general consensus was that 'the disease has disappeared before civilisation'. The flip side of this argument was that plague 'has returned with a country's decline and barbarism'. Milroy specifically targeted the Ottoman Empire: 'Wherever the Ottoman dominion has prevailed, civilisation and social improvements have retrograded rather than advanced.' He further claimed that 'pestilential epidemics' were bound to recur in 'Syria, of Turkey in Europe and Asia, and of the Barbary states', as their hygienic condition remained poor. This was particularly true for the 'residents upon marshy alluvial soils near the Mediterranean or near certain rivers, as the Nile, Euphrates and Danube; the dwellings being low, crowded and badly ventilated; a warm moist atmosphere; the action of putrescent animal and vegetable matters, unwholesome and insufficient food; and great physical and moral wretchedness'. Others would point to the Libyan Merdj highlands around Benghazi and Derna, particularly among the local

Bedouins. To Milroy, 'the recently instituted Board of Health at Constantinople' should not believe the illusion that they saved Istanbul from 'an invasion of the plague for some years past exclusively and entirely to the establishment of lazarettos and quarantine restrictions there'.[15] Rather, they should take to heart the warning Lord Posonsby had given them at the beginning of their efforts.

The Ottomans remained committed to a contagionist programme of preventing plague. After its establishment in 1838, the Ottoman Quarantine Administration stopped all boats going through the Straits to check if they came from a contagious port. If the boat in question did, they would have to spend the requisite time in quarantine. Questions of whether or not there was a case of plague on board or in the port of origin were thus more important than the boat's hygienic or sanitary situation. The Ottoman authorities would also take other contagionist measures to protect Istanbul from outbreaks in the countryside. In February 1839, for example, 'the Sublime Porte sent an imperial edict to the judges, notables, and dignitaries of Anatolia', which stated that a land cordon would be set up around the six districts surrounding the Ottoman capital on its Anatolian side. The decree also instructed local judges, notables and dignitaries to respect the institution, and to obey its police, engineers and other officials.[16] This followed the example of the Habsburg Empire, which had established a permanent land cordon along its southern border with the Ottoman Empire to prevent plague and cholera in the late eighteenth century.

The Ottomans were also largely in control of both the Constantinople Superior Health Council and the Quarantine Administration. The Constantinople Superior Health Council, which agreed to take on foreign members, was almost always chaired by an Ottoman. The minutes of the Council itself were written in Ottoman Turkish, with only a small French summary at the end of each session.[17] Ottoman subjects dominated the Quarantine Administration leadership, including the General Secretary, the Supervisor of Military Affairs and the Chief of the Domestic Sanitary Police. The Ottoman authorities selected and trained lower-ranking Quarantine Administration officials, who were sent out to smaller stations at Beirut, Smyrna, Crete, Erzurum and Trablusgarp (Libya) for further training. The Ottomans also recruited Europeans for the Administration, but they were subject to the same rules and regulations as their Ottoman counterparts.

The Ottomans did not hesitate to use these institutions in order to project their power internationally. In 1846, the Istanbul quarantine 'successfully implemented precautionary measures' to protect itself from a plague outbreak in 'Egypt, Syria, Benghazi, Tripoli, Marseilles and southern Italy'. During the outbreak, Muhammad Ali, the great moderniser of Egypt, came to Istanbul to pay homage to the sultan. Ahmed Midhat Efendi (1844–1912), a renowned

Ottoman scholar and later head of the Ottoman Quarantine Administration (1894–1908), related in his history of the Ottoman quarantine that Muhammad Ali also came by boat 'in order to see the importance the Sultan gave to public health'. Ironically, the Ottoman Quarantine Administration stopped his boat in Smyrna. Officials there considered the boat suspect, as it had come from 'plague-ridden Egypt'. Muhammad Ali waited in the city eight days before quarantine officials from Istanbul arrived to inspect and disinfect the boat.[18] The fact that a widely acknowledged international dignitary who had threatened to take over the Ottoman state himself over the past twenty-odd years had to await 'disinfection' helped the Ottoman quarantine gain broader respect from a domestic audience used to a seemingly endless stream of defeats; from the French invasion of Egypt in 1798, to the Greek rebellion of 1821–9, and Muhammad Ali's Syrian campaigns of 1833–8.

The Ottoman Quarantine Administration sought to bolster this support further when it declared that, contrary to Clot-Bey's and Aubert-Roche's findings, 'the incidents of plague that did occur in Syria, Anatolia, and elsewhere in the Empire always came from the outside'. Thus, 'plague was not endemic in . . . any of the Imperial Ottoman domains'.[19] Ahmed Midhat further ridiculed Clot-Bey's and Aubert-Roche's focus on 'prophylactics – a peculiar science – which ignored the truth about effectively implementing quarantines'.[20]

The Ottomans would face their first great challenge after the Clot-Bey and Aubert-Roche report in 1858–9, with the outbreak of plague among the nomads of Benghazi. Foreign observers, such as Radcliffe and the French scholar Joseph-Désiré Tholozan (1820–97), claimed that the outbreak infected 10,000 in fifteen months, 4,000 of whom perished.[21]

Dr Bartoletti, an Ottoman member of the Constantinople Superior Health Council and long-time Imperial representative to the International Sanitary Conferences, was dispatched to the province on 3 June 1858 'to help local officials stop the spread of the disease'.[22] He found that only 200 had contracted the disease, and thirty had died. He further stated that the outbreak was spontaneous and of a contagious nature, and should not be blamed on the Bedouin's nomadic lifestyle, their dwellings, burial customs or even peculiarities of the soil. To him, the plague was connected to a famine that had weakened the resistance of the local population to the disease, and had nothing to do with the climate *per se*. Why, he asked, should one 'ever pretend that the plague originated from the Sahara, the Libyan desert, or the Sudan, for to my knowledge the high temperature in that region appears to be an insurmountable natural obstacle to the disease [just like it is] . . . in Upper Egypt'.

The measures Bartoletti and other local quarantine officials implemented also contradicted Clot-Bey's and Aubert-Roche's infectionist views. The province of

Benghazi was declared from the beginning of the epidemic to be under a foul bill of health, and was placed under strict quarantine to prevent maritime contact with other ports: 'The strictest surveillance was exercised on deliveries from suspected vessels [from the Libyan coast] to the Dardanelles in order to guarantee the capital of the Empire.'[23] Bartoletti complained that the foreign councils in Benghazi and Tripoli tried to interfere with these measures, and he brought up the matter at the Constantinople Superior Health Council upon his return: 'In that meeting they decided that the assembly would be the sole authority for public health affairs when it came to the provinces and that consuls did not have the right to intervene . . . The Sublime Porte has the sole power to confirm and implement the assembly's decisions.'[24]

Dr Laval, a French doctor, and Dr L. Arnaud, a Frenchman in the Ottoman Quarantine Administration, challenged Bartoletti when they investigated a later outbreak of plague in Benghazi in 1874. They found that the disease was in fact endemic among the nomadic population of the region. They attributed the outbreak to their poor hygiene, the burial of their dead and, above all, to the pestiferous nature of the soil when dampened after years of drought. Laval formed an ad hoc committee including the American Consul General in Tripoli as well as two Maltese doctors and several notables from Benghazi. After writing a letter to the Ottoman governor of Benghazi begging for greater hygienic measures, Laval fell ill and died from plague, prompting Arnaud to follow up his efforts. Arnauld established sanitation camps for the afflicted, fed and clothed the patients and had them go through a decontamination process. He praised the Ottomans for trying to alleviate the population from the famine, but drew attention to the inadequate measures they had taken. In effect, he called for a belated embrace of infection as the cause of plague and for an end of Ottoman denials that the disease was endemic in parts to the area.

QUARANTINES AND COMMERCE

Such differences of opinion can also be seen in relation to the transport of goods through quarantines. Ahmed Midhat mentioned: 'Quarantines were involved in commercial competition for a while. Some states would implement quarantines needlessly and this hindered international trade. The merchant marines of each country complained about this.'[25] He and other Ottoman Quarantine Administration officials claimed that the system could be implemented without inhibiting free trade. Bartoletti took a similar line at the first International Sanitary Conference in 1851 that: '[Europe] should adopt as extensive a quarantine system as possible to protect public health, but not disrupt international commerce. The Turkish quarantine is an example of how this may be done.'[26]

The British, the Ottoman Empire's leading commercial partner until the 1880s, disagreed profoundly with these views.[27] Dr John Simon wrote in 1865 that a quarantine was 'a mere irrational derangement of commerce'. To him, a quarantine subordinated commercial to political interests, and ensured that 'a community lives apart from the great highways and emporia of commerce'.[28] Sir Arthur Helps, the Chief Administrator of the British Quarantine Administration in 1869 wrote despairingly:

> It might be advisable to keep up regulations as regards quarantine which you could not at all justify medically, but which you could justify commercially and internationally, seeing that our commercial marine would be smitten by most severe regulations in other countries if we did not keep up quarantine here.[29]

Milroy focused on the role of cotton, the chief British export from Egypt during the nineteenth century. Unsurprisingly, he cited the Clot-Bey and Aubert-Roche report. He posited that while a plague 'epidemic raged at Alexandria [in 1835] among the servants and employees living in the magazines of the Egyptian government', roughly 100,000 bales of cotton were exported to Europe without any ill effects. Plague may have been on board eight of the sixteen British vessels laden with 31,709 bales of cotton, 'yet their cargoes did not prove more dangerous than those of the non-infected vessels'. No person was 'infected in consequence' even though there were no precautionary measures to disinfect 'this immense quantity of an article that has always been deemed highly susceptible of retaining the infectious effluvia'. This case proved Clot-Bey's and Aubert-Roche's conclusion that 'there is nothing to prove articles of merchandise can transport the disease beyond epidemic foci'.[30]

These anti-contagionist arguments resonated in the International Sanitary Conference of 1851. Dr P. Segur-Dupeyron, a member of the French Royal Academy of Medicine and French Consul in Damascus submitted a report on the subject of plague and merchandise after conducting exhaustive archival research and inspections of Mediterranean quarantine facilities. He found only 'a single event where plague was transmitted through goods': a case in Istanbul where 'a porter named Mehmet Huseyin caught it from infected luggage in the lazaretto of Kuleli'. He concluded 'that there was no positive evidence that plague was transmitted by infected merchandise . . . especially cotton'.[31] The British and French delegates supported these findings.

They were in the minority, however. Dr Rosenberger, a member of the St Petersburg Superior Health Council was the first to weigh in on the side of the Ottomans:

> A third of my honourable colleagues agree with the British who are not afraid that the plague would be spread by vegetable or animal matter. But are not you who oppose contagion imposing another theory on us that is to the detriment of public health? The majority of physicians believes in contagion and denounces the new theory. There are a number of cases where vegetable and animal matter transmitted plague. I have seen this myself in Odessa in 1837 and in Sevastopol in 1829 and 1830. Dr Bartoletti who has the most personal experience of us all will tell you that vegetable as well as animal matter can pass the plague and that it is impossible to recognise whether or not it came from an infected place. These experiences prove that prudent measures are in order. I trust the older regulations – drawn up after centuries of experience and detailed registration – far more than the people today who make false arguments. As seen recently in Turkey, the adoption of stringent quarantine regulations was a brilliant success.[32]

Bartoletti then successfully proposed that a ship laden with cotton, flax and hemp with a poor bill of health begin quarantine 'only after the cargo is completely unloaded'.[33] As a result, the conference final report categorised cotton, hemp and linen as liable to possible quarantine. The majority of participants also dismissed 'the findings of Segur-Dupeyron since he did not physically observe the lazarettos nor properly inspect the cotton bales'.[34]

The prospects for the British and French improved once the construction of the Suez Canal began in earnest in the 1860s. Although the issue was not resolved in the International Sanitary Conference of 1866, most observers quickly realised the enormous amount of traffic that would go through the Canal and that the Zone – although internationally run – could possibly be subject to quarantine as well. The next International Sanitary Conference in Vienna in 1874 specifically broached this topic. The majority of participants accepted that each country could choose between 'quarantine' and 'medical inspection' as a precautionary measure to prevent plague or cholera. Those that maintained contagionist quarantine practices – like the Ottoman Empire – promised to 'diminish its stringency as heretofore practiced'.[35] Henceforth, the British adopted 'the state of health of those on board . . . [as their] guiding principle . . . [and not] the arrival of a ship from an infected country'. To them, quarantines were outmoded as 'the period of incubation of this sickness onboard became the standard or limit of the duration of detention'.[36] This meant in effect that the British and the anti-contagionist majority on the Suez Canal International Sanitary Board could ensure the free flow of traffic by adopting 'medical inspection' instead of 'quarantine' procedures.

CHALLENGES TO THE CONSTANTINOPLE SUPERIOR HEALTH COUNCIL

Ottoman quarantine officials continued to face a number of challenges to their authority. One of the most profound was the controversy over how to fund the institution. When Mustafa Reşid Pasha, one of the chief architects of the Ottoman reform movement, met in 1840 with the foreign powers to discuss how the Ottoman quarantine could be internationalised, he reached an agreement about taxation: 'Foreign states would have the right to send one delegate a piece to the quarantine assembly . . . [but] foreign boats [like Ottoman ones] would pay a special public health tax.'[37] The rate was fixed at 40 piastres per boat regardless of size or number of passengers. But as early as 1842, Ottoman officials worried that this tax alone could not pay for their quarantine system. Baki Efendi, the chief financial official for the Ottoman quarantine wrote a memorandum to the Sublime Porte that the 5,660 piastres raised between March 1840 and February 1841 could not pay for even one-tenth of the total expenses. He feared that 'they would shut down public health stations inside the Ottoman dominions – including coastal stations'. He proposed that passengers on ships – including foreign vessels – pay 1 piastre each as a public health tax.[38]

The Ottomans raised this issue again at the 1851 International Sanitary Conference in Paris. After arguing that the uniform tax of 40 piastres per boat was too low for commercial vessels Bartoletti persuaded the participants that:

> The taxes the authorities took from commercial boats were not sufficient to cover public health expenses. The conference decided that the authorities should receive a suitable amount of revenue and that the taxes should be levied according to the tonnage size of each boat instead of small amounts based on official receipts.[39]

The Conference agreed in theory that foreign boats above 50 tons would pay 3 piastres per ton and Ottoman boats in the same category would pay 2 piastres per ton. Any boat weighing 50 tons or less would pay 1 piastre per ton, and smaller incidental taxes on passengers and their goods would also be allowed. The foreign participants asked for five months' delay to get their respective countries consent, but did not respond.[40]

By September 1862 the Ottomans proposed to reduce the tax:

> They suggested that two liras be taken from boats up to fifty tons; five liras from boats between fifty-one and 200 tons; and ten liras from boats larger than 200 tons; twelve liras from steamers regardless of tonnage if they were penalised.

> If the boats came from contagious locations without a bill of health they should undergo quarantine twice.[41]

The British – who had the largest tonnage of commercial vessels in the Ottoman waters – complained in 1866 that the Ottoman quarantine was overstaffed, overpaid and could reduce the number of its offices. Nonetheless, the Ottomans did eventually implement a renegotiated rate in 1872: 'Every boat 500 tons or below would pay 20 piastres as a base rate. Others would pay additional fees beyond the 20 piastre base rate; 12 piastres additionally for those above 500 tons; and 8 piastres from those above 1,000 tons'. The Ottomans and the foreign powers also agreed to form a 'mixed committee' to discuss any changes to the rates.[42]

The Ottoman quarantine officials also had to struggle with the British and the French during two significant outbreaks of cholera. The first case occurred during the Crimean War, when the British, French and Sardinians sent their fleets to Istanbul. The French Marshal Saint Arnauld refused to undergo quarantine and British complained that public health regulations caused military delays. The Ottomans retorted that 'even battleships should be subjected to quarantine', but in April 1855 they allowed 15,000–20,000 French Imperial Guards to camp at the Davut Pasha Barracks.[43] 'Cholera soon broke out among them . . . [and] a severe epidemic followed'. Cholera spread from the camp to 'Pera and to those villages on the Bosporus the nearest to the cholera focus'.[44] The Constantinople Superior Health Council met multiple times during the next ten months, quarantining the soldiers to limit the outbreak. They also constructed separate foreign cemeteries for the French and British, and implemented new burial and butcher shop regulations. Some of the foreign officers continued to disrespect the Ottoman authorities, 'arguing that they came from disease-free countries'.[45]

A new cholera outbreak in 1865 spread throughout the major ports of the Ottoman Empire. Bartoletti, the representative of the Ottoman quarantine authorities, spoke at the International Sanitary Conference convened in Istanbul in 1866 to discuss the outbreak. He found that the cause of the epidemic could be traced to Egypt in at least two cases. Infected passengers from the Egyptian frigate *Moukbiri Sourur* spread the disease in Istanbul after the captain falsely declared that there was no case on board. In Smyrna, a vessel arrived from Alexandria with a foul bill of health, and cholera spread to the city after a patient was brought to the lazaretto. Bartoletti also claimed that the Ottomans were proactive in handling the disease, as they quarantined over 25,000 people at various stations throughout the eastern Mediterranean and Black Sea. There were only 480 confirmed cases of cholera, 238 of whom had died.[46]

Others were highly critical of Bartoletti's account. An international inquiry about the case questioned the low number of cholera cases in the Ottoman lazarettos, and claimed on the basis of foreign consular reports that there were many more unreported deaths in the towns and surrounding villages. They posited that 2,500 died from cholera in Smyrna, while only nine died in the city's lazaretto. Similarly, nearly 350 died in the villages surrounding the Dardanelles and only fifteen died in their lazaretto. They suspected that the lazarettos themselves helped to spread the disease:

> See how things happened at the Dardanelles. From the beginning of July, many cases of cholera had been admitted to or developed in the lazaretto, when on the twelfth, a soldier of the guards, at the gate of the establishment, was attacked by the disease. He was transported to the neighbouring hospital, where he rapidly sank. On the next day, eight cases of cholera occurred; namely, two among the soldiers of the guard at the gate of the lazaretto, three in the garrison of the fort adjoining the establishment, one in the town, distant an hour's walk by land, but much nearer [to] the sea, in the person of a *garde de sante*, who had left the lazaretto two days before, one in another quarter of the town in an individual who went every day to the lazaretto to sell cakes, and finally one in the person of a boatman of the Health Office. This was the point of departure of the epidemic which developed itself in the town, and did much mischief there.[47]

This case led to further questions about how the Ottomans might have been covering up the actual extent of the epidemic:

> It would be a matter of the greatest interest to be able to say precisely in what matter things have happened at each [of the Ottoman ports]; but the want of precise information does not permit this. It is easy to understand, also, how many interests are opposed, in most of these cases, to the exact truth being known.[48]

This point leads to the conclusion that the Ottomans needed to open up their quarantine to greater foreign scrutiny. Despite this criticism, the Ottomans refused to surrender authority over ports on their own sovereign territory.

Criticisms of the Ottoman quarantine regarding plague also continued throughout the second half of the nineteenth century. Dr Armedee Latour, a member of the French Consultative Committee on Public Hygiene complained in 1878 that the Ottoman quarantine officials lacked the training and resources to carry out the task:

> The reports by the Central Administration of sanitary doctors along its coast and provinces are largely incomplete, and show a lack of competence and concern. One doubts that the sanitary doctors are qualified for such a mission. It is difficult

to obtain qualified people in such remote countries, as they have very little resources. [The Ottomans] were forced to assign individuals who are not trained or certified. The quality of their medical personnel has gradually improved in recent years, but the majority of the Ottoman Administration is very narrow-minded, believing that they are carrying out their task when they show that the disease does not exist.[49]

To Latour, fighting the plague effectively meant implementing sanitation measures throughout the Empire, and not limiting their efforts to maritime quarantines stations: 'The Sanitation Administration in the Ottoman Empire . . . should be such that the plague cannot escape the vigilance of their agents in the smallest village'.[50] Dr J. D. Tholozan, a member of the Epidemiological Society of London and the Medical Academy of Paris likewise judged:

> Even if we accept the hypothesis that we can eliminate plague germs by establishing sanitary cordons and quarantines, it is feasible only in theory. In practice it is not so as seen in Cyranique [Benghazi]. Can one disinfect the nomads of Benghazi? The Ottoman Empire simply does not have the means to carry out such a task . . . It does not have the army, police, and financial resources to do so.[51]

These critics were also bitter that the Germans had begun to support the Ottoman Quarantine Administration – just like the Austrians and Russians did. Dr Adrien Proust (1834–1903), a long-time French participant at the International Sanitary Councils, claimed a German colleague delegate to Constantinople Superior Health Council supported an Ottoman protest that increasing foreign pressure exposed 'the country to disease'.[52] Tholozan was similarly disgruntled about Dr A. Hirsch, a German representative to the 1874 International Sanitary Conference who discounted the Benghazi outbreak, and claimed that the last plague epidemic in the Ottoman Empire occurred in Constantinople in 1842.[53] Dr A. Fauvel, long-time Inspector General of the French Sanitary Service feared that it was impossible for the European powers to develop a unified policy towards the Orient, 'as they are divided by antagonism, jealousy and struggles over influence'.[54]

Proust suggested in 1897 that the European governments should try to use their influence to reassert control over the Constantinople Superior Health Council: 'The foreign consulates should dominate, and have a commensurate number of representatives. This is especially urgent in . . . Constantinople, as a lack of action would result in serious disadvantages.'[55] Without foreign domination, 'the Council is bound to remain, like the Ottoman government, ultra-quarantine in doctrine'.[56] To him, the Europeans should try to accomplish what they had already done in Alexandria:

> Alexandria's Council underwent a fortunate change in 1892, since the number of Egyptian members outside of the President have been reduced to three. They are appointed by the government and do not have a right to vote in the event of a tie in the committee. Beforehand it was composed of nine Egyptian members. Now the Council has become an international body since the local element has been reduced. Additionally, a Permanent Committee has [been] substituted for the President when urgent decisions need to be made. No one attached to the Egyptian government or Maritime Company has been considered.[57]

In contrast, he accused the Ottomans of unfairly 'possessing effective supremacy in a council that should be international':

> In short, Ottoman civil servants have successfully attacked the Sanitary Council of Constantinople every day and weakened its authority. The Council represents sanitary interests of the first order and its ruin might affect the health of Europe's trade and navigation. The Turkish government would determine all sanitary measures if that were the case.[58]

In his opinion, the Ottomans had an effective majority in Council, as eight of the twenty-one voting members represented the Sublime Porte, and four to six more were non-Muslim Ottoman subjects, who voted with their countrymen even though they were appointed to represent other foreign governments. He called a reorganisation of the Council:

> By reducing the number of Ottoman members from eight to four and make the American, Persian, Dutch, Spanish, Belgian, Swedish and Norwegian governments send their own citizens. Without it, the Council is bound to remain, like the Ottoman government, ultra-quarantine in doctrine.[59]

The Ottoman government, however, successfully avoided Proust's plot in 1897 and continued to hold sway in the Council, much as it did from the 1840s onwards. Thus, the Ottomans were able to assert authority in the face of political threats, financial crisis and the outbreak of epidemic disease. Seemingly nothing could force them to re-evaluate their contagionist emphasis on quarantines, lazarettos and governmental control of their coastline.

THE SUEZ AND THE HAJJ

It is therefore quite striking that the British, French and other European powers should succeed in radically changing international rules concerning quarantines and plague in the 1890s. They continued to see plague and other epidemic diseases as primarily infectious, but they now acknowledged the need to hold infected and infectious people and cargo in quarantine when need be – as sometimes was the case if they came from a non-European country. This development primarily involved establishing quarantines stations around the Suez Canal, which the British *de facto* controlled as part of the protectorate it had declared in 1882. The British, French and Dutch successfully petitioned during the International Sanitary Conferences to develop more stringent policies regarding the Hajj pilgrims – all in the name of preventing outbreaks of plague and cholera. These policies also coincided with imperialist interests as they were already attentive to anti-colonialist movements in Egypt, India and Java. The colonial powers were very concerned that the pan-Islamic Ottoman Sultan Abdul Hamid II (1876–1909) might use the annual Muslim pilgrimage to Mecca and Medina to mobilise this opposition for his own political purposes.

Although there were serious concerns raised about the pilgrimage to the Hijaz during the cholera outbreak of 1865, quarantines along the Suez Canal Zone were not finalised until the 1892 International Sanitary Conference in Venice. Thereafter, large British-dominated quarantines were authorised at Moses Wells by the Mediterranean entrance to the Canal to deal with southbound vessels, and at Djebel Tor at the opposite end in the Red Sea for northbound boats, along with smaller satellites at Abou-Saad, Abou-Ali and Vasta. While the Ottomans had also established stations at Kamaran for boats headed to Jeddah, and Bab-el-Mandeb for pilgrims from the Indian Ocean heading towards the Red Sea, the Suez quarantines were more important as all maritime traffic passing between the Mediterranean and Red Sea were under its jurisdiction.

In the International Sanitary Conferences of 1894 and 1897 a series of new regulations about cholera and plague were implemented about the Suez. European vessels that had a clean bill of health were given immediate practique without any restrictions or requirements. Other European vessels were to be placed under a five-day observation after passing through the Suez as long as none of their third-class passengers disembarked and the boat had a disinfection chamber and adequate medical staff. Non-European vessels – even those going to the pilgrimage – could be granted similar terms if the country that owned the boat adhered to the convention. The Suez Quarantine Authority, however, had the ability to detain any non-European vessel if there were cases of plague or cholera in the Hijaz that year and make them go through a special disinfection procedure:

> The pilgrims shall be landed; they shall take a shower bath or bathe in the sea; their soiled linen and any portion of their personal effects or their baggage, open,

> in the opinion of the sanitary authority, to suspicion, shall be disinfected. The duration of these operations, including disembarkation and embarkation, must not exceed seventy-two hours.[60]

The pilgrims would then be dealt with by the quarantine authorities, who often gave inoculations of anti-plague or anti-cholera serum. The Haffkine anti-plague vaccination produced high fever in the patient within hours of the shot; and, as Ottoman quarantine official Besim Ömer related, sometimes up to 5–10 per cent of those vaccinated died in the process.[61]

Other regulations were targeted towards 'risk groups'. Poorer pilgrims were heavily discouraged from making the journey, and were prohibited from boarding a pilgrimage vessel without a return ticket. First- and second-class passengers were given more lenient treatment, especially if the boat carried few or no people in third-class. Third-class passengers would also face greater restrictions and surveillance when in quarantine. Those ship-owners who could not provide adequate steamboats, food, water, medical equipment and staff would not be allowed to make the journey. Those that did would be subject to additional scrutiny from the port of embarkation.

Disinfection procedures were extended to medical inspection and fumigation for rats and rodents in 1897, but it did not lead to a fundamental reworking of the 1894 regulations, which were first drawn up before Alexander Yersin's discovery of bubonic bacilli in Hong Kong.

Critics of Ottoman contagionist measures were delighted with the new procedures. Proust lauded the new surveillance facilities and procedures:

> The Suez Canal is of immense importance to maritime relations throughout the Mediterranean basin. The pilgrim must be subjected there to complete disinfection before arriving in Mecca . . . The disinfection methods they practice are necessary given what happens on board the pilgrim ships. As Dr Ferrari, the director of the Suez Health Service, makes the authoritative judgement that 'pilgrims are always transported in rundown ships'. Pilgrims excessively crowd the boats, and there is no free space left. They always number more than the bill of health indicates for the sanitary authorities of the Hijaz. A number of times the ships have lacked tents to shelter the pilgrims on the bridge, meaning that they are exposed to sunshine all day long. Water and food are also insufficient and very expensive. The information the captains and doctors give about the ships are often very inaccurate. Ferrari adds: 'I have often received certificates from the captain and the border officials saying that the pilgrims are in perfect health. But when I pay them a medical visit I notice the sick dying in the middle of filth without any medical assistance from the doctor or the border officials.'[62]

The Ottomans had no easy answer to these developments. They initially stood by their own contagionist rules and regulations, but they, the Greeks, the Serbs and the Portuguese, were the only participants to the 1897 International Sanitary Conference not to agree to the new convention. They also would not be able to internationally licence their doctors or provide adequate disinfection chambers unless they adopted 'medical inspection' and other prophylactic methods. Continued Ottoman intransigence would marginalise their influence in international sanitary policies and threaten their maritime links with the distant province of Hijaz. The Constantinople Superior Health Council soon called on new hygienic measures to survey the pilgrimage in the light of these new realities.[63]

Muslim dissatisfaction with the Suez quarantines grew, however. İbrahim Rifat Paşa (1857–1936), an Egyptian general who to helped lead the annual sultan's procession to Mecca and Medina in 1903 complained of his treatment at Djebel-Tur on his return journey. He and the entire procession were forced to undergo quarantine there for sixteen days because one of the pilgrims who accompanied him allegedly caught the plague. Their 'medical inspection' was brutal:

> A group of Christian Greeks were responsible for the inspection. Some treated our possessions well, but others turned over all our pots and poured out the contents, and then threw them on the ground. The majority [of the items] were perfume bottles and delicate silver pots, most of which were damaged . . . A lot of things, especially the expensive and valuable ones were stolen . . . They [then] forced us to go into the bath houses, and made us wear dark, loose cotton clothes without buttons. We left the bath houses with bare heads and feet and waited in the heat of the sun and musty air . . . We caught diseases, and had head colds and chest pains during this time . . . They gave us tin pots to use both for drinking water and for cleaning the toilets . . . The toilets were not cleaned every day and the flies gathered horribly. How is this healthy?[64]

Rifat Paşa protested to the Egyptian Interior Minister, but he was told that he and the other members of the procession had no choice but to comply.[65]

CONCLUSION

Istanbul was also hard-pressed by such complaints. The Empire's quarantine officials could not do very much about maritime passage through the Suez, as their sovereignty over Egypt and the Canal Zone was practically non-existent. Ottoman access to the Hijaz was also largely limited to sea traffic, as pilgrims much preferred steamers to the old caravan routes. Those who did take a caravan were vulnerable to robbery from local Bedouins. Muslim pilgrims, particularly Arabs from Egypt, Palestine, Syria and Iraq voiced their opposition to British domination, but also sensed the pending colonisation of the region.

The construction of the Hijaz Railway, inaugurated in 1903, partially solved this problem. Pilgrims from the Empire, Europe and western Russia would have a viable alternative to using the sea lanes after its completion. This would also take the pressure off the Ottoman government to fully give in to international pressure, since they would exercise their own sovereignty over the routes. Yet the Ottomans would not abandon their newly found faith in prophylactics and medical inspection, as this could be used to help further consolidate their control over the distant province. The government could indeed implement public health reform by increasing its policing powers to regulate buildings, sanitation, water supply and medical facilities. There would be growing opposition to such measures by local interests who wished to limit this intrusion. The Bedouins would resist such efforts, vandalising newly constructed waterways in much the same way they tried to sabotage the new railway.

The Ottomans had come nearly full circle. When they established the quarantine in 1838, they followed standard European practices. Their action, however, provoked the European powers – particularly the British and the French – to declare that sanitary measures, which did not interfere with free trade by implementing government control, were far more effective in combating plague. These measures allowed the British and French to consolidate their economic and political hold on Egypt, which transformed over the nineteenth century from an Ottoman province to a European colony. This is best symbolised by the European takeover of the Suez Canal in 1869. Some thirteen years later, after the declaration of the country as a British protectorate, the Europeans were able to take over Egypt's public health institutions. By the 1890s, the British and other European powers, increasingly aware of an anti-colonialist backlash against them in Egypt and elsewhere in the Islamic world, decided to use the quarantine facilities established at the Suez to regulate those Muslims going through the Canal Zone on their way to the annual pilgrimage to Mecca. The result was a series of rules and regulations which discriminated against the pilgrims, defining Europeans as hygienic and civilised, and Muslims as poor and unsanitary. Some Muslims believed that they were being humiliated much in the same way as the poor captive patients who Clot-Bey and Aubert-Roche had subjected to experiments for their seminal 1846 study that had defined infectionism in the first place. The Ottoman quarantine authorities now sought to embrace these same infectionist methods but use them for their own ends.

NOTES

1. Ahmed Midhat, 'Devlet-i aliyye-i Osmâniye', pp. 96–7.
2. Milroy, *Quarantine and the Plague*, pp. 13–14.
3. Milroy, *Quarantine and the Plague*, p. 12.
4. Milroy, *Quarantine and the Plague*, p. 13.
5. Milroy, *Quarantine and the Plague*, p. 14.
6. Milroy, *Quarantine and the Plague*, p. 15.
7. Milroy, *Quarantine and the Plague*, p. 22.
8. Milroy, *Quarantine and the Plague*, pp. 22–3.
9. Milroy, *Quarantine and the Plague*, pp. 23, 26–7.
10. Milroy, *Quarantine and the Plague*, p. 38.
11. Milroy, *Quarantine and the Plague*, pp. 31–2.
12. Milroy, *Quarantine and the Plague*, p. 57.
13. Milroy, *Quarantine and the Plague*, p. 57.
14. Anonymous, *Plague*, p. 43.
15. Milroy, *Quarantine and the Plague*. pp. 25–7.
16. Ahmed Midhat, 'Devlet-i aliyye-i Osmâniye', pp. 95–6.
17. Ahmed Midhat, 'Devlet-i aliyye-i Osmâniye', pp. 102–4.
18. Ahmed Midhat, 'Devlet-i aliyye-i Osmâniye', p. 5.
19. Ahmed Midhat, 'Devlet-i aliyye-i Osmâniye', pp. 102–4.
20. Ahmed Midhat, 'Devlet-i aliyye-i Osmâniye', pp. 96–7.
21. Anonymous, *Plague*, p. 21; Tholozan, *Histoire de la Peste Bubonique*, p. 247.
22. Ahmed Midhat, 'Devlet-i aliyye-i Osmâniye', p. 112.
23. Dr Bartoletti, 'La Peste de Benghazi', pp. 11, 15.
24. Ahmed Midhat, 'Devlet-i aliyye-i Osmâniye', pp. 112–13.
25. Ahmed Midhat, 'Devlet-i aliyye-i Osmâniye', pp. 108–9.
26. International Sanitary Conference, *Procès-verbaux de la Conférence Sanitaire Internationale Ouverte en Paris le 27 Juillet 1851*, p. 235.
27. Jan Erik Zürcher, *Turkey: A Modern History*, pp. 76–90.
28. Anonymous, *Plague*, pp. 59–60.
29. Anonymous, *Plague*, p. 46.
30. Milroy, *Quarantine and the Plague*, pp. 52–3.
31. International Sanitary Conference, *Procès-verbaux (1851)*, pp. 313, 399, 347.
32. International Sanitary Conference, *Procès-verbaux (1851)*, p. 333.
33. International Sanitary Conference, *Procès-verbaux (1851)*, p. 424.
34. International Sanitary Conference, *Procès-verbaux (1851)*, p. 419.
35. Anonymous, *Plague*, pp. 46–7; 58–9.
36. William J. Simpson, *A Treatise on Plague*, p. 352.
37. Ahmed Midhat, 'Devlet-i aliyye-i Osmâniye', p. 98.
38. Ahmed Midhat, bid. 'Devlet-i aliyye-i Osmâniye'p. 101.
39. Ahmed Midhat, 'Devlet-i aliyye-i Osmâniye', pp. 108–9.
40. Ahmed Midhat, 'Devlet-i aliyye-i Osmâniye', p. 111.
41. Ahmed Midhat, 'Devlet-i aliyye-i Osmâniye', pp. 115–16.
42. Ahmed Midhat, 'Devlet-i aliyye-i Osmâniye', pp. 117–19.
43. Ahmed Midhat, 'Devlet-i aliyye-i Osmâniye', pp. 109–11.
44. International Sanitary Conference, *Report to the International Sanitary Conference from*

a Commission from that Body to which were Referred Questions Relative to the Origin, Transmissibility and Propagation of Asiatic Cholera, pp. 76–7.

45. Ahmed Midhat, 'Devlet-i aliyye-i Osmâniye', pp. 109–11; International Sanitary Conference, *Report*, pp. 76–7.
46. International Sanitary Conference, *Report*, pp. 28, 68–76.
47. International Sanitary Conference, *Report*, p. 71.
48. International Sanitary Conference, *Report*, p. 71.
49. Joseph-Désiré Tholozan, *La Peste en Turquie dans les Temps Moderns: Sa Prophylaxie Défectueuse, sa Limitation Spontanée*, pp. 198–9.
50. Tholozan, *La Peste en Turquie*, pp. 192–3.
51. Tholozan, *La Peste en Turquie*, p. 205.
52. Adrien Proust, *La Défense de Europe Contre la Peste et la Conférence de Venise de 1897*, p. 265.
53. Tholozan, *La Peste en Turquie*, p. 202.
54. Tholozan, *La Peste en Turquie*, p. 196.
55. Proust, *La Défense de Europe Contre la Peste*, p. 264.
56. Proust, *La Défense de Europe Contre la Peste*, p. 266.
57. Proust, *La Défense de Europe Contre la Peste*, p. 263.
58. Proust, *La Défense de Europe Contre la Peste*, pp. 265–6.
59. Proust, *La Défense de Europe Contre la Peste*, p. 266.
60. League of Nations, *Report of Commission to Inquire into International Arrangements regarding Epidemic Disease Prevention in Certain Areas of the Near East (Basin of the Eastern Mediterranean and Black Sea) and in Connection with the Mecca Pilgrimage*, pp. 34–5.
61. Ömer, 'Veba-Ta'un', p. 236.
62. Proust, *La Défense de Europe Contre la Peste*, pp. 238–40.
63. Proust, *La Défense de Europe Contre la Peste*, pp. 267–8.
64. İbrahim Rifat Paşa, *Mir'atü'l Harameyn bir Generalin Hac Notları*, pp. 449–51.
65. Rifat Paşa, *Mir'atü'l Harameyn bir Generalin Hac Notları*, p. 566.

CHAPTER

7

PLAGUE, SANITARY ADMINISTRATION AND THE END OF EMPIRE

INTRODUCTION

The Ottomans had fully embraced a new vision of plague and quarantines in the wake of the 1894 and 1897 International Sanitary conferences. This vision of disease indeed accepted Alexander Yersin's 1894 discovery of the bubonic plague bacilli in Hong Kong as valid for justifying hygienic measures that sought to eliminate the ultimate cause of the disease: the filthy, unsanitary living conditions of 'unmodernised' societies. The only way the disease in question could be defeated was through governmental action. This meant establishing a sanitary administration that would not only establish hospitals to treat the sick through vaccinations and other modern treatments, but also constantly police the impoverished and marginal. As seen in the previous chapter, the Europeans after 1838 often saw Middle Eastern Muslims – particularly the people of Egypt – as the uncivilised bearers of infectious disease. Such a view helped to support the long-term British and French aim to colonise the country, given the implication that only the Europeans were civilised enough to establish an effective sanitary administration of the area.

The Ottomans, convinced by developments towards the end of the century – the establishment of the European-dominated Suez Canal in 1869, the British defeat of Urabi Revolt and the establishment of a protectorate in 1882, and the International Sanitary Regulations of 1894 and 1897 – had now decided to adopt an infectionist view of plague and other epidemic diseases.

A 1908 Ottoman imperial edict declared that they could not limit their activities to policing ports and the docks, granaries and storehouses connected to them through the maritime quarantine. The government was also now empowered to inspect, repair and rebuild sewers and even private homes: 'Above all we must get rid of the filth that allow rats into a city.'[1] This meant above all to police the poor:

> Patients who have come down with plague are to be sent for quarantine to prison-like cells for solitary confinement. Their clothes and undergarments will be destroyed or put inside metallic boxes encased in solution . . . [Their houses must also] be emptied . . . The houses should be burned along with their furniture if they are of little value. Their prior inhabitants should be sent far away and examined in tent-hospitals. There their goods would be subject to disinfection procedures. [Even if the houses are of value], no one can live [there] for two months; the municipal or state government will have to provide a place for the inhabitants to live.[2]

These measures were implemented in urban areas throughout the empire. Hospitals, vaccination centres, sewers, plumbing and building codes were, of course, established in Istanbul – the capital of the empire, which over the course of the nineteenth and early twentieth centuries was filled with recent Muslim refugees from the wars that bedevilled the Balkans and Caucasus.

Yet an even more remarkable effort was made in the Middle Eastern provinces, particularly Ottoman Iraq and the Hijaz, where the policing efforts involved social and religious groups that historically were only partially integrated into the Ottoman state.

Iraq was of growing international importance. Its southernmost province of Basra was envisioned to be the terminal station of the famed Berlin to Baghdad Railway, a project which would have allowed both the Ottomans and their German sponsors to bypass the Suez Canal by a new rail route. The Ottomans and Germans, as well as their British rivals, were also increasingly aware of Iraq's untapped petroleum resources – vital to nearly every aspect of the industrial age. The railway, begun in 1903, was only in its initial stages of construction, and the Ottomans sought alternative means to try to consolidate rule in the distant province. These efforts were complicated by the Shiites of the region, who travelled to southern Iraq each year on an annual pilgrimage to the holy cities of Najaf and Karbala. The Ottomans, perhaps fearful that their local Shiite minority would become increasingly restive in their desire to unite with their numerous foreign co-religionists, called on sanitary measures to control the incoming Shiite pilgrims – especially from Persia.

The Ottomans were also greatly concerned with the Hijaz, the western Arabian province that was home to the two holiest cities of the Islamic world, Mecca and Medina. They faced growing criticism by foreign observers that plague was running rampant there. One British physician noted hundreds of deaths from plague in outbreaks between 1906 and 1908 and urgently called for international action to stem further outbreaks.[3] His criticism was painful, given the geopolitical realities of the time. Britain, having declared a protectorate over Egypt and the Suez, had nearly complete naval dominance over the Red Sea and eastern Mediterranean. British influence was bound to grow, especially in the Hijaz port cities of Jeddah (64 km from Mecca) and Yanbu al-Bahr (164 km from Medina). By 1900, the Ottomans felt compelled to embark on another railway project – the Hijaz Railway – to link the province by rail to the rest of the empire. The British and other European powers repeated their earlier concerns about the threat of epidemic disease, especially as it related to the annual Muslim pilgrimage. The Bedouins of the province were also worried that the railway would diminish their incomes, as they collected annual subsidies from the Ottoman government and fees from the pilgrims for providing goods and safe passage. While the Ottomans completed the Damascus–Medina stage in 1908 and planned to extend the railway to Mecca, they also sought other means to consolidate rule in the cities of the Hijaz: the sanitary administration.

The leading Ottoman sanitary administrative official for both of these projects was Kasım İzzeddin (1858–1926). From 1894 until 1912 İzzeddin was involved with the quarantine and sanitary efforts in Mecca, as well as in Baghdad and Basra, and was appointed to a variety of posts during this time, including Inspector General of the Ottoman Sanitary Administration, Director of the Hijaz Sanitary Administration and Chief Sanitary Officer of the Quarantine at Baghdad, Basra, Damascus and Sinop. It was no accident that the bulk of these posts were in the Arab provinces of the Ottoman Empire. İzzeddin was a Lebanese Sunni Muslim, very much concerned that his home province, like Palestine, Syria and Iraq faced the threat of colonisation by the British and the French. Such feelings were revealed in the 1911 International Sanitary Conference held in Paris, where he, as Ottoman representative, raised the issue of religious equality. If a sanitary administration was necessary for the Muslim pilgrimage in the Hijaz on the principle that such meetings of pilgrims from faraway places could introduce new epidemic diseases, he asked, why should sanitary administration not be necessary for every pilgrimage? Thus, in his opinion, the Ottomans should run a sanitary administration not just in the Hijaz for Sunni Muslims, or in Najaf and Karbala for Shiite Muslims, but also in Jerusalem for Jewish and Christian pilgrims. He followed this up with arguments to tighten international restrictions on vessels approaching Ottoman ports in the eastern Mediterranean from 'infected ports' – which would allow the Ottomans to medically inspect and detain boats of Jewish immigrants and pilgrims from Russia.[4] Although İzzeddin's effort to change the regulation was unsuccessful, it was likely appreciated by other key Ottoman sanitary administrative officials, such as Ruhi Al-Khalidi (1864–1913), a leading Arab Young Turk supporter from a prominent Palestinian family, who was one of the first to call attention to the increasing Zionist presence in his homeland. Khalidi's insistence that the newly-created Hijaz Sanitary Administration be directly controlled by the Ottoman central government through the Interior Ministry was also a telling moment. Khalidi, like İzzeddin, invested his hopes in centralising rule in the region, since the Ottomans then would be even more committed to retaining sovereignty in the north-eastern Arab provinces, as they linked Anatolia to both Iraq and the Hijaz.[5] Opposition to the sanitary reforms carried out by İzzeddin would be quite sharp, particularly on the part of local Shiites and Bedouins.

The British had a very curious reaction to these developments. Dr Frank G. Clemow, the British Representative to the Constantinople Superior Health Council and the Crown's Delegate to the 1911 International Sanitary Conference, often applauded İzzeddin for adopting an infectionist understanding of plague and other epidemic diseases, and supported many of his sanitary reforms. These reforms would often involve new technologies, such as water supply and fumigation, that would potentially increase Ottoman dependency on London for both finance, technological know-how and even energy dependence on coal supplies. His attitude, like that of the British Empire, would only change during the First World War, when the British cut their support and started to foment rebellion among the Shiites and Bedouins.

The following chapter will examine the continuing dialogue İzzeddin and Clemow had on sanitary reform in both Iraq and the Hijaz from the beginning of the twentieth century until the outbreak of the First World War, and detail the consequences of the reforms during and after the ensuing conflict.

THE OTTOMAN SANITARY DEFENCE OF IRAQ AND THE PERSIAN GULF

İzzeddin was not the first Ottoman sanitary official to face serious challenges on the Empire's eastern frontiers with Persia and the Gulf. The Ottomans had first set up quarantine stations to prevent the spread of plague and cholera after the 1851 Paris International Sanitary Conference. Ottoman officials had argued that epidemic diseases often passed into the empire through Persia, as witnessed by the 1831 plague outbreak there. Further epidemic outbreaks of plague and cholera occurred throughout the 1860s and 1870s, and Ottoman and Persian officials often blamed each other as the first country to have the disease. Dr Bartoletti, who represented the Ottoman Empire at the International Sanitary conferences in the decades before İzzeddin took office, accused the Persians in

1871 of turning a blind eye to plague cases in their country. He thought that a land cordon should be set up along the Ottoman–Persian border, and helped to supervise the establishment of two main stations at Khanikin, along the main southern Persian road to Baghdad, and at Bayazid in the mountainous north. He and the Ottoman government believed that the main carriers of the disease were the northern mountainous nomads and the Shiite pilgrims who made an annual trek to the holy cities of Najaf and Karbala, and also nearby Baghdad.[6] Representatives of the Persian authorities, such as Tholozan, the founder of the Persian Sanitary Council in 1868, claimed that the Ottoman nomads of northern Iraq were to blame for outbreaks of plague and cholera. In his opinion, the Ottomans should cease their criticisms, and the needless land cordon, and work to improve sanitary conditions among the nomads instead.[7]

The Ottomans also set up two key maritime quarantine stations in the region after 1851. The first was at Basra, the southernmost Ottoman port in Iraq, and also at the Hormuz, key to controlling access to the Persian Gulf. Indian Shiite pilgrims to southern Iraq – also declared a high risk group for plague and cholera – justified the existence of these stations even into the first decade of the twentieth century. The 1903 Sanitary Convention directed that all ships entering the Gulf be subjected to medical inspection at Hormuz. Those entering the Ottoman Empire had to undergo a second inspection at Basra: any vessel which had previously docked at a port with confirmed cases of plague or cholera was required to complete five days observation before being allowed to go.[8]

Yet it was only during İzzeddin's time that these arrangements fundamentally changed. İzzeddin and the Ottoman government set the tone when, under international pressure, they abandoned the quarantine station at Hormuz. Clemow claimed that British-run alternative quarantine stations in the Gulf 'rendered wholly unnecessary any special clauses in the conventions for the sanitary defences of the Persian Gulf'.[9] This shift revealed Great Britain's near total maritime domination of the Gulf.

İzzeddin thus limited his efforts to the Basra, Khanikin and Bayazid stations. Of these three, Basra was the most inconsequential. Between 1903 and 1913, an average of only 3,334 people entered the Ottoman Empire at Basra, compared with an annual average of 42,031 entering the Ottoman Empire from Persia.[10] The Khanikin station alone processed about two-thirds of the Persian traffic to the Ottoman Empire. The station also played an important financial role, since they charged a sanitary tax of 10 piastres for every Shiite pilgrim who crossed the border. The bulk of the foreign pilgrims were Persians, although a significant number of Russian Shiites also passed.[11]

The greatest controversy concerning the pilgrim traffic revolved around the pilgrims' tradition of burying their deceased loved ones at Najaf and Karbala.

The Ottomans had generally restricted the practice to only those 'dry' corpses that had mummified, since they suspected 'fresh' corpses of transmitting plague and cholera. The only exception to this rule was the bodies of those who had died only twelve hours prior to crossing the border. The Ottomans collected a sanitary tax of 50 piastres per corpse, five times that for a live pilgrim. This resulted in a substantial amount of income, as evidenced by an annual average of 3,900 bodies taken across the border at Khanikin between 1909 and 1914.[12] These numbers peaked in 1912–13, when, under İzzeddin's supervision, the Ottomans collected taxes on a record 7,558 corpses.

The tax was controversial. Clemow, for instance, dismissed Ottoman concerns that the bodies might spread disease:

> While disease has been repeatedly introduced and spread by the movements of the Shiite pilgrims, it is noteworthy that it has apparently never been so by the movements of the Shiah corpses. No instance could be traced in which either plague or cholera – the two diseases mainly dealt with under the international conventions – had been imported or diffused by these dead bodies.[13]

Clemow suspected that local Ottoman officials were seeking to exploit the pilgrims for their own monetary gain, as seen in his own description of the practice in Najaf:

> On arriving in the outskirts of Najaf the bodies are first deposited in a small enclosure, or morgue, built in the desert near the town. Here the taxes are collected; the bodies are removed from their outer wrappings or coffins, and placed in large coffins belonging to the *defnieh* department (the nature of which will be defined shortly). The other wrappings and coffins are burned by the health officials, in the desert near the morgue. The commission was consulted as to the necessity of continuing this system of incineration. The *labad*s or *shibna* – that is, the shrouds around the coffins – are of considerable value, and the wood of the coffins would be precious in these regions, where trees are unknown and all wood has to be imported. The local authorities were anxious for permission to arrange for the preliminary disinfection of the coffins, which they then proposed to sell; the revenue thus obtained would, they claimed, enable the local health assembly to put up a steam disinfecting stove, in which the shrouds also be disinfected and afterwards sold. Some such form of disinfection was attempted a few years ago, but it led to serious abuses and was abandoned. The commission definitely condemned a return to the former system. The practical difficulties in the way of properly disinfecting a large number of coffins and shrouds would be considerable, and, for obvious reasons, incineration is the only proper fate of such objects.[14]

The pilgrims and the local Shiite population subverted the Ottomans by propagating a 'sanitary contraband in dead bodies':

> It is not rare for corpses to be brought secretly, at night, accompanied by armed bands of Arabs or Kurds, numbering some scores or even hundreds, who buried corpses in the cemetery outside the town without any formalities being complied with. Such contraband will always exist, for it could only be met by using armed forces superior to the others, and in each instance many lives would probably be sacrificed. Contraband in fresh (and dry) bodies was largely exercised by persons in the holy cities who made a profession of the practice. It seems that all the principal towns in Persia and Mesopotamia had representatives or commissioners in the Shiah cities; they were generally gravediggers, muleteers, *khan*-keepers [shopkeepers], *khadims* [pilgrim-guides], and even *sayyids* [descendants of the Prophet] and *ulemas* [Islamic theologians]. The bodies were addressed to such commissioners, who would go out into the desert to meet them and give the bearers of false certificates, testifying that death had occurred within the 12-hour zone.[15]

Clemow thus recommended that the Ottomans focus on the live pilgrims alone as the main concern of their medical inspections.

Moreover, he also drew attention to the poor hygienic state of affairs in Ottoman Iraq. Besides pointing out the endemic nature of the Tigris and Euphrates river valleys as their damp soils often caused putridity and disease among the houses and settlements there, he highlighted the need for better sanitary measures in central and southern Iraq. He remarked that 'there [were] no drains in Karbala or Najaf'. Most of the houses had cesspools and, in his opinion, 'it [was] not surprising that many diseases are rife in [these] cities'.[16] To him, Basra was also highly problematic, as water supply for this town of 50,000–60,000 people was directly from nearby creeks contaminated by surface pollution. There was no municipal drainage system, and this muddied the unpaved streets with sewage.[17]

Basra was also in dire need of modern building codes. The city's 'sunburned and kiln-burned brick' houses were in bad repair. They were allegedly also badly ventilated and overcrowded. Some dwellings even had strange underground cellars:

> In all the larger houses are found underground chambers, or *serdabs*, where the inhabitants may escape from the great heat of the summer; many are forty or fifty, and some even eighty or 100 feet below the ground. If reports be true, these cellars are often the scenes of unspeakable vices.[18]

İzzeddin largely concurred with Clemow on the need for sanitary reform in these cities. After being assigned as the Chief Sanitary Officer of Baghdad in 1905, he established a main office in that city, as well as the major towns of Najaf, Karbala and Kiazimein. Satellite branches were also established at Ali-El-Gharbi, Amara, Bugheila and Gourna on the Tigris, and Kufa, Museyyib, Samawa and Shenafieh on the Euphrates. They were staffed by sanitary doctors, police and administrative officials under the supervision of the Ottoman Interior Ministry and the Constantinople Superior Health Council.[19] İzzeddin did not just 'report to Constantinople [on] the appearance of plague or cholera in their district', and enforce the tax codes and regulations on the pilgrims and the traffic in corpses, as Clemow supposed. He also established major hospitals and enforced new housing regulations in Baghdad, Najaf and Karbala.[20]

İzzeddin also agreed with Clemow that poor sanitary conditions often involved lawlessness. For instance, he blamed the notables of Najaf and Karbala for their involvement in the contraband trade in corpses. He also was concerned that the influx of poor pilgrims from Persia disturbed genuine pilgrims.[21] This revealed a new attitude among the Ottoman authorities towards outbreaks within the realm. Enacting sanitary policing measures led to social discrimination against the poor and religious discrimination against non-Sunni Muslims.

İzzeddin was frustrated by budgetary and logistical concerns, however. The Ottoman government was forced to foot most of the bill for the sanitary reforms, since the Constantinople Superior Health Council – a nominally international body – could not use the income from the Shiite pilgrim taxes without the consent of its foreign members. Getting up-to-date equipment for the projects, and bringing in sufficient numbers of engineers and construction crews, was also a problem since the railway project was nowhere near to being completed – it remained some 563 km away from Baghdad in 1918, long after İzzeddin's service in Iraq had ended.[22]

Nevertheless, İzzeddin did manage to worsen relations with the local population. Local Shiites and pilgrims resented higher taxes and regulation. This was often aggravated by the fact that a number of the medical officials were non-Muslims hired from abroad. Lamec Saad, a German-born quarantine official who worked at the Khanikin border station in the early twentieth century, was accused by one Persian Shiite who complained that: 'We are Muslims and not infidels. We do not want to go in quarantine and pay the money.'[23] This complaint much recalled that of İbrahim Rifat Paşa, the Egyptian general who protested at the humiliation of Sunni Muslim pilgrims by Greek doctors at the Tor quarantine by the Suez Canal. Such humiliations prompted action against the quarantine and the government who ran it. The only difference was that this time the Ottomans were on the receiving end, an ominous sign for rebellion in the years ahead.

SANITARY REFORMS IN THE HIJAZ

Issues about quarantine, medical inspection and sanitary administration was be on a much greater scale in the Hijaz. This was reflected in the 1911 Paris International Sanitary Conference, where İzzeddin and Clemow represented the Ottoman and British sides, respectively. The Ottomans and British sought to reach accommodation on several key issues; first and foremost, how the Conference's sanitary regulations related to the Hijaz Railway project. The Hijaz Railway greatly concerned the British after 1908, since it allowed pilgrims from the Empire and beyond to bypass the British sanitary controls at the Suez Canal. Clemow and his government feared that the annual number of 12,000–20,000 pilgrims that used the route could spread cholera and plague to the Hijaz, elsewhere in the Ottoman Empire, Europe and beyond if adequate medical inspection facilities were not implemented along the route. Austro-Hungarian, French, Dutch and Italian delegations shared the British concerns since they, too, had many Muslim colonial subjects of their own who used the route. Yet the Ottomans firmly resisted any formal international sanitary control over the railway. As Ali Mukhtar Bey, İzzeddin's fellow countryman, related at the Conference: 'The Ottoman government considers the Hijaz Railway as an interior line and does not believe it is more dangerous than rail lines found in other countries.' Clemow and the majority of the Conference conceded that the Ottoman Empire had the right to run its own sanitary administration within the borders of the country.[24]

This quick approval was the result of a joint Ottoman–British effort to achieve international consensus on the subject. The British sought to influence Ottoman policy on the Hijaz Railway and the Ottomans needed to get Great Britain's consent to use sanitary tax revenues to develop a sanitary administration in the area. İzzeddin began this cooperation in 1908 when he helped form a joint ad hoc committee with Clemow to select a new quarantine station on the railway line. Clemow and the other foreign powers agreed to fund the effort temporarily, pending discussion at the Conference. They set up their temporary quarantine at Medain-i Salihi, a town roughly 350 km to the north of Medina. The Ottomans recommended the site as it was situated on the northern border of the Hijaz, and would thus fit well within current administrative divisions. İzzeddin, the committee and the local Ottoman sanitary officials established a makeshift medical camp, and work was done to supply food, water and shelter to the 12,933 pilgrims who were inspected that year at the station for plague and cholera. Cholera was diagnosed in 101 pilgrims, fifty-seven case of which were fatal. İzzeddin felt that despite improvisations, awkward planning and occasionally mismanaging these infections the mission was ultimately successful, as 'the disease did not spread [from the Hijaz] to Syria'.[25]

Clemow raised doubts about choosing Medain-i Salihi as the permanent site of the railway quarantine. He argued that the water supply to the town was too poor and was very vulnerable to sandstorms – factors that forced the committee to establish the quarantine 10 km away from the railway, causing further delays for the travellers. He was also worried about resistance from local Bedouins to reforms. He saw this firsthand when: 'On the day of our arrival there was a serious attack made on the head of the [rail] line and in the fight which followed some forty Bedouins were said to have been killed.'[26] To him, the Bedouins' resistance to the quarantine stemmed from their belief that the Prophet Muhammad himself had forbidden outsiders to stay in the town:

> Medaini Salih is, to those Muslims who know the legend that gives it its name, more or less under a ban . . . As far as can be gathered the legend is not known to the bulk of the pilgrims and it did not apparently lead to any overt objection on their part to the choice of Medaini Salih for the temporary lazaret in the last two seasons. Possibly it might not lead for many years to come to any difficulties in connection with a prominent lazaret here. But there would always be the risk of its doing so someday. Pilgrims in any case admit unwillingly to a quarantine, and should any fanatic among them choose to recall the legend (which is referred to frequently in the Koran) and incite the other pilgrims to rebel against being quarantined here, a very serious condition of affairs might be brought about. It might easily become impossible to force the pilgrims to remain here and quite possibly they would take the law into their hands and destroy the buildings. As it is intended to spend large sums in installing the new lazaret, it would be foolish to run this risk, more particularly as the transfer to another side of a lazaret, once built, is as costly (indeed it would practically mean) its rebuilding anew.[27]

Clemow argued that the Ottoman quarantine station should instead be established in Tebouk, a town also on the Hijaz Railway roughly 283 km north of Medain-i Salihi. He believed that the town had a much safer water supply, better quarries and was less prone to sandstorms. He also argued that the quarantine station at Tebouk could be established much closer to the railway than at Medain-i Salihi. In his opinion, the place was also a strategic location, as the Bedouin tribe, Beni Attiyeh, had a good working relationship with the Ottoman authorities there.[28]

İzzeddin concurred. He agreed that water could easily be brought to the Tebouk station and did not foresee any great administrative difficulties for the Ottoman sanitary administration. Although he did not explicitly mention the issue of the Bedouins, he was no doubt aware that the Bedouins around Medain-i Salihi violently protested the quarantine station out of fear that the government would soon interfere with their tribal affairs.[29] From İzzeddin's viewpoint, moving the station to Tebouk would cause fewer possible complications, as the Bedouins there were much more amenable to the increased governmental presence.

The Ottoman quarantine station was quickly constructed in Tebouk the following year in accordance with Clemow's recommendations. İzzeddin noted that in 1909 there were only three cases of cholera seen in Tebouk and that the disease again did not spread to Syria.[30] Clemow and İzzeddin had basically worked out an arrangement on the Hijaz Railway station before they arrived at the Conference. İzzeddin would follow Clemow's instructions on how and where to establish the station, but the Ottoman sanitary officials would run it, partially funded by the sanitary taxes. The Conference merely ratified this arrangement.

The Ottomans also faced considerable pressure from the Europeans to make sanitary reforms in the major towns of the Hijaz, particularly Mecca and the adjacent Red Sea port of Jeddah. Proust complained about Jeddah after 1894 that:

> One should note the filthiness of the town. The Ottoman government does not take responsibility, as pilgrims who disembarked from [the Ottoman quarantine at] Kamaran are crowded into rooms of more than thirty people. Garbage was strewn throughout the streets, and then never cleaned. The government collects municipal taxes of fr.175,000 per year but no work is done.[31]

Proust saw İzzeddin's efforts at that time to send professional medical teams, restore water pipes and build fumigation stations in Jeddah, construct a 1,400-bed guest house and three hospitals in Mecca and clean the streets of Medina as laudable, but ultimately unsuccessful.[32] In May 1895 'local Bedouins' assassinated Abdur-Razzack, the British Vice Consul for Pilgrimage Affairs in Jeddah, and wounded the British, French and Russian consuls in protest at the measures.[33] Thereafter the municipal sanitary workers neglected their duties and the local Muslims of Jeddah allegedly polluted the new water supply when they performed ablutions and washed their linen.[34]

İzzeddin himself conceded that his early efforts were not enough. He agreed that the local municipal government could not handle these efforts on their own, as 'epidemic diseases occur during the pilgrimage', affecting far more than just the provincial population. The locals also did not have either sufficient funds or capable officials to administer the reforms. He documented this with a May 1910 report from Zihni Pasha, the Ottoman Governor of the Hijaz to the Ottoman Interior Ministry. The Governor mentioned that Hussein Bin Ali (1854–1931), the Sharif of Mecca, could only raise 50,000 paistres as sanitary tax, and that nothing more could be expected from them or the local Bedouins whom he represented:

> Everyone is thirsty and hot, both during the pilgrimage – when the blessed die – and during the off-season [when the region] is continually crowded with more than 100,000 people. [The Hijaz] is truly a gathering place for the entire Islamic world, no matter what time. Only the Ottoman state can maintain order for the Muslim pilgrims who come from every end of the earth. It must do so with its funds and personnel as agriculture and industry do not exist, and trade is limited.[35]

In İzzeddin's eyes, the Ottoman government should assume direct control since state treasury funds would be involved. In fact, the Ottoman government approved a budget of 3,184,703 paistres – roughly comparable to that of the Hijaz Railway.[36] It expended 1,275,280 paistres from the central treasury to pay for the sanitary reforms, a far higher amount than the 50,000 paistres taken from local taxes, or even the 130,000 paistres it raised from foreign pilgrims. The government's fiscal commitments underscored its claim that the reforms were its holy duty: 'The administration of the pilgrims' sanitary affairs is incumbent upon the exalted government and the Islamic Caliphate.'[37]

İzzeddin and his co-administrators elaborated these arguments when they launched the Hijaz Sanitary Administration in 1910:

> The Hijaz Sanitary Administration is providing great service to the Islamic world. There is no doubt that the people who have died in the Hijaz surpasses many times over the casualties of great battles . . . Consequently, it is necessary for the Hijaz Sanitary Administration to undertake such a holy duty to help the sick, like the wounded on the battlefield . . . It is natural that the number of pilgrims will increase as long as we protect their health and well-being. If we do so, Muslims will joyously come here to fulfil their sacred duties. We will be rewarded for this in the next world . . . We have a responsibility to the more than 300 million Muslims of diverse nations and tribes who gather here in brotherhood. We need to advance their health, social and economic well-being, and show the superiority of Islam. This would demonstrate how knowledge, civilisation and the economy could be used to achieve God's will. But how is that possible when 100,000 Muslims come here without food, drink, shelter, and are unprotected and unclean? In short, they lack sanitary precautions and thus help spread contagious disease. The building of more residences for the pilgrims worsens the situation. Only the Hijaz Sanitary Administration can address these problems and gradually improve living conditions.[38]

The new administration embarked on a variety of reforms, including the establishment of sanitary police and engineers, medical personnel, permanent hospitals, tent-hospitals, pharmacies, fumigation stations, administrative buildings, shelters for poor pilgrims, new sewage, water supplies, and new building and food regulations for all four major cities in the Hijaz (Mecca, Medina, Jeddah and Yanbu).

The Hijaz Sanitary Administration had now become another branch of the Ottoman central authority. İzzeddin, the Director of the Hijaz Sanitary Administration, worked in the name of Talat Pasha (1874–1921), the Interior Minister, much like the Director of the Hijaz Railway did. The directors of the Hijaz Sanitary Administration and the Hijaz Railway both tended to clash with Hussein, the Sharif of Mecca, whom İzzeddin ironically thanked for running the Jeddah sanitation efforts prior to his arrival. His dismissive attitude towards Hussein's municipal authorities – the local notables and Bedouins – was telling. New regulations required Hussein not only to obey İzzeddin as the Director of the Hijaz Sanitary Administration, but also to send him an annual report on how İzzeddin's reforms were implemented in the province.[39]

İzzeddin and Clemow discussed sanitary measures in Jeddah in some detail, particularly regarding the establishment of new hospitals and water supplies. The European powers paid great attention to Jeddah, since it was the major port of the region, and, as such, had the strongest foreign presence. Clemow complained that Jeddah's one working hospital was 'quite inadequate to the needs of the place':

> There is a small municipal hospital situated inside the wall that completely surrounds the town on its eastern side and not far from the Mecca gates. It is a one-story structure built against the town wall. It contains two wards for twelve and eight patients respectively; the wards have no flooring, their floors being a beaten earth. Close by is a wooden shed in bad condition used for dysentery patients; it is almost entirely without furniture. In brief, this hospital – though those in immediate charge of it have apparently done their best with limited means placed at their disposal – is altogether too small and too primitive for a town like Jeddah, with its vast floating population. The inspection commission in its report consequently urges the Turkish government to build a large general hospital capable of 150 or 200 patients and suggests a suitable site where it might be built.[40]

İzzeddin apparently received far harsher criticism from other foreign officials:

> There was . . . no hospital in Jeddah, except for the city hospital, which foreign embassies complained about numerous times. One stated: 'The Jeddah hospital is

> only a single wooden barrack. There are no hospital attendants, food or water. It has wooden stumps for beds, with holes in it for the patient to relieve themselves. For this reason, human excrement has piled up on the floor. The place is like a dunghill. Your patients suffer from various diseases like smallpox and dysentery. The place simply spreads disease among the patients'. The Consul sent a picture of the hospital where six patients – three with smallpox – were lying down on a wooden stump. There also was a picture of a funeral of a man who died a day ago. The procession was covered with flies, and one could see the human excrement under the wooden stumps.[41]

İzzeddin worked quickly to address these concerns. Two hospitals, one a 100-bed military barracks facility, and the other a forty-bed tent-hospital were established within the first year of the Hijaz Sanitary Administration.[42] İzzeddin's success in establishing the hospitals without incident was remarkable given the assassination of Abdur-Razzack in 1895 in protest against fumigation stations that were erected in the city.[43]

The establishment of new water facilities in Jeddah proved to be more difficult. The city had suffered a drought in 1906, when Clemow had inspected the facilities. Water in Jeddah at the time he visited was basically limited to rain water, which individuals in Jeddah had collected in tanks and cisterns throughout the city, and numerous wells which had been dug near the city walls. The water from both of these sources was extremely poor in quality, and quite unhealthy to drink – especially the brackish well-water. There were four other springs outside the city, but only one of them, Ayn Bariman, was able to provide the city with any water. Ayn Bariman's water was carried 'by petroleum cans on the back of a camel or donkey'. The other three springs, Ayn Farraj, Ayn Hamidiye and Ayn Veziriye, had water pipes to the city, but they were constantly sabotaged.[44]

Clemow cited local opposition against water supplies as the main obstacle to reform. He suspected 'certain citizens of Jeddah', [who] own the majority of the water tanks', were the ones actually behind the Bedouin attacks. Led by local notables like 'Hadrami – a very influential man who opposes all efforts made in order to improve the situation', these interests had damaged the water pipes in an attempt to retain their monopoly over the cistern water and the Ayn Bariman springs.[45]

Clemow proposed establishing water-distilling machines to process local well and rainwater. This would alleviate the need to rely on the local cistern interests, and would avoid the nearly impossible task of securing pipelines to the wells outside the city – since they would remain vulnerable to attack. Though the distilling machines were presumably safe behind the guarded walls of the medical facilities, the Ottomans were still wary of further opposition:

> Vested interests are extremely strong; the owners of tanks will do all they can to prevent the sale of distilled water, if they do not actually attack the machines. The people themselves, strongly conservative by nature, will take time to get accustomed to distilled water in place of the other waters they have been used to drinking. In time, however, there should be no question of the distiller or distillers, under proper management, yielding a handsome annual profit. This aspect of the question is, however, in truth, one of secondary importance in comparison with the real necessity, on sanitary and humanitarian grounds, of providing Jeddah with a certain, abundant, and safe water supply.[46]

Clemow felt, however, that popular suspicion of the distilled water could be overcome in time, especially given its higher quality and cheaper price. He cited his own government's success in establishing a similar machine in Oman, where the locals fought over the distilled water once they had tasted it.[47]

İzzeddin followed up on Clemow's suggestions by buying a water distiller (100 tons per day), and a large ice-maker (2,000 kg per day), along with the electrical cables and equipment to run both machines.[48] He also accessed a new water source only 5 km to the north of Jeddah to supply the distillation and ice machines. They were secured within his sanitary compound.[49] Much of the city celebrated:

> In January 1329 [1911], they completed installing the ice machines and electricity generators [in Jeddah]. The government officials held a ceremony with the consulates of the foreign powers, local notables and steamboat agents. They slaughtered rams and prayed that the Caliphate of Islam's glory may be increased. They also wished for the prosperity of the Hijaz Sanitary Administration. The opening day of the ice and electric generators was a joyful one for the people of Jeddah. They opened the doors of the factory to the public and all the people around came to see the machines and were happy.[50]

Such successes were key to convincing both the foreign powers and the local population that the Hijaz Sanitary Administration's programme of social and political centralisation was there to stay. Yet foreign support – particularly that of the British – was vital. İzzeddin had followed Clemow's suggestions on nearly every matter brought to him – be it for the railway quarantine station or Jeddah's hospitals and water supply. İzzeddin also imported the distillation and ice machines from Great Britain over naval routes largely controlled by Great Britain. The coal he required in Jeddah to provide the electricity for the machines also had to be shipped in – as this bulk good could not be brought overland since the railways from Medina to Mecca and Jeddah were not complete.

Unsurprisingly, the British even suggested that the Ottomans use Cardiff coal instead of domestic coal from Zonguldak on the Black Sea coast. The British claimed that the coal burned cleaner and provided more energy.[51]

Yet the celebratory scene over ice in Jeddah, reminiscent of similar festivities for the Hijaz Railway,[52] conveyed sovereignty in a concrete way that the pilgrims and the local population were bound to appreciate. The Ottomans under İzzeddin sought to further express this sovereignty in the district through their new-found social disciplinary powers as medical and sanitary inspectors.

Poverty, in İzzeddin's opinion, was a 'difficult social disease for the holy pilgrimage' that bred epidemic disease, and degraded the sanitary and moral climate for everyone in the region. Two beggars had allegedly begun a cholera outbreak in the Hijaz after travelling from Mecca to Medina on foot in 1909. They were not the only ones who caused problems, according to İzzeddin. Poor pilgrims, who numbered approximately 20 per cent of Muslim visitors, often 'began begging and annoying other pilgrims after arriving in the Hijaz' by going from Jeddah to Mecca with their bowls:

> They infringe upon the health of the pilgrims and do things which spread disease. When the diseases abound, there are twice as many dead among them than among the other pilgrims. These people do not come to the Hijaz in order to perform the pilgrimage . . . You cannot call them by the title Hajji. They do not deserve the respect the real pilgrims do.[53]

İzzeddin's first initiative to deal with the problem apparently ended in failure:

> When we formed the Mecca Sanitary Administration in 1312 [1895] we tried very hard to ameliorate the situation for the beggars. We brought them to our hospitals and gave them food and clothing but this did not satisfy them. Instead, the beggars began to act in a hostile manner. They did not know what goodness means. They pretended to be sick and wanted money from those who passed. They did not like it when the Sanitary Administration picked them up from the streets and sent them to the hospitals.[54]

When İzzeddin used a former barracks to house the poor pilgrims after he became General Director of the Hijaz Sanitary Administration in 1910, the beggars continued to resist. Münir Pasha, the Commander-in-Chief of the Hijaz Division, informed him that: 'None of the poor pilgrims wanted to stay in the former barracks, saying that it was very far away from the city and the holy places . . . But the guesthouse was only two kilometres away [from the city centre].'[55]

İzzeddin approved of measures the Europeans had taken at the 1894 Paris International Sanitary Conference. The French, Austro-Hungarians and Dutch strongly supported travelling restrictions, as all three had substantial Muslim colonial populations. Proust, the main French delegate to the conference, 'mentioned that only 60 per cent of the Muslims from Java, 50 per cent of Bosnian pilgrims and only a few thousand French pilgrims returned home'. The Austro-Hungarians, no doubt influenced by the fact that up to one-third of the Bosnian Muslim population had left for the Ottoman Empire after the 1878 occupation,[56] sought to use an internal passport system for the pilgrims. The Dutch followed suit by closely examining returning pilgrims with local Javanese Islamic authorities. If the returning pilgrim could not pass a 'test' about his visit, he was subjected to a monetary penalty.[57]

The British also tried to restrict the traffic of their Egyptian pilgrims as much as possible. As Clemow related:

> An Egyptian desirous of making the pilgrimage must secure a special passport from the Mudir of his district or the governor of his town. This passport contains a detailed description of the individual and spaces for receipts for quarantine fees and caution money deposited by the pilgrim. The man must then visit the sanitary inspector of his district, who satisfies himself that the passport is in order, so that he will be able to identify the individual on his return. Later, the passport must be signed by the passport officer at Suez on his outward journey, who again satisfies himself that all is in order before embarkation. On his return journey the passport officer at Tor forwards the document directly to the sanitary inspector of the pilgrim's district. On emerging from Tor the pilgrim is given a voucher which enables him to land at Suez and he is then instructed to proceed direct to his home and present himself daily to the sanitary inspector who at the end of seven days hands back to him this passport duly signed in order that he may be able to withdraw his caution money from the local authority. This system may sound a little complicated but it works extremely well in a country where the people are accustomed from time immemorial to obey the orders of the government officials.[58]

Nevertheless, the British were reluctant to adhere to international regulation of Indian Muslims, as this would imply outside interference in their own internal affairs. They thus referred the question to the Ottomans, saying that they would agree to the restriction only if 'the Sultan, acting as the Caliph, [ordered] that no one should go to Mecca from any part of his Empire without obeying this rule'.[59] The Ottomans, represented at the 1894 conference by Turhan Pasha, maintained that poor pilgrims should not be hindered from performing their religious duty. Nevertheless, Turhan Pasha was willing to refer the question to his government for further consideration, since Islamic legal scholars had conflicting positions on the topic.

İzzeddin, the Ottoman Delegate to the 1911 Paris International Sanitary Conference, reversed the previous Ottoman position: he now supported forcing pilgrims to purchase a return ticket prior to their departure to the Hijaz, as well as pressuring wealthy Muslims who sent substitutes to perform the pilgrimage to provide adequate money for the journey. İzzeddin also advocated greater policing measures once the pilgrims reached the Hijaz, since 'leaving the poor pilgrims who came to do their sacred duty on the streets is contrary to Islam and the Caliphate'.[60] Quarantine officials were to medically inspect the pilgrims before and after arrival, and sanitary police made sure that pilgrims were clean. They also would keep 'beggars' off the streets, and inspect the pilgrim's food and accommodations.[61]

İzzeddin's discriminatory statements about the poor in the Hijaz and the policies he took towards them confirm similar sentiments he had shown in Iraq. Acting as a leading sanitary administrative official, İzzeddin made a major departure from earlier Ottoman views on the plague and other major epidemic diseases. He showed that the Ottomans were now willing to use existing social divisions to further their own governmental power.

Yet İzzeddin's sanitary policies conflicted with the local population just as much as they did with poor foreign-born pilgrims. Clemow spoke of this issue when he talked about the spread of plague in the Hijaz in 1907:

> It is a remarkable fact that, with the single exception of a fatal case of plague in a Javanese pilgrim, the outbreak in Jeddah has been strictly confined to the native inhabitants of the town . . . I am inclined to attribute this relative immunity to the fact . . . that most of [the pilgrims] live in homes specially built for the purpose, which are surveyed, cleansed and whitewashed and put into order before the arrival of the pilgrims; and that those who are too poor to stop in houses camp out in the open air, where they are little exposed to the infection of the plague either from contact with the inhabitants of the town or with rats.[62]

Clemow blamed the local Arabs for resisting the sanitary reforms:

> There seems to have been much difficulty in applying measures for the suppression of the outbreak. The Arab inhabitants dreaded European interference more than the disease; the large majority of cases have only become known to the authorities after death and it is certain that many that recovered were brought to the knowledge of the latter. Scarcely any of the cases have been removed to hospital. When a death from plague has become known the house where

> it occurred has been disinfected . . . Shortly after the revival of the disease in January it was proved beyond a doubt that rats were dying from plague and were in all probability the main channel by which the infection was being spread. Small rewards, of the value of one penny, were offered for the bodies of dead rats, but there is no evidence at present that this measure led to any substantial results. The medical staff of the town was strengthened and an ample supply of prophylactic was furnished to them, but the latest reports showed that it was almost impossible to induce the people to allow themselves to be inoculated. In some cases the opposition to the authorities took a more active form and violence was used. In one case a native woman – possibly interpreting too literally the injunction to keep coals of fire on the other's head – poured a torrent of hot ashes from a window onto the head of a disinfector who attempted to enter the house.[63]

Clemow implied here that the only solution to the problem was to use the sanitary police and a centralised command structure to enforce the reforms – exactly the same path that İzzeddin followed some three years later when he created the Ottoman sanitary administration.

Still, İzzeddin sometimes ran into difficulties even with his strong institutional presence in the region. This was particularly clear when he tried to regulate the sale, butchering and disposal of sacrificial rams, which the pilgrims bought annually at Mena on the outskirts of Mecca:

> The problem in Mena is due to the slaughtering of rams and the overcrowding of the streets. The pilgrims stay in Mena for only three days, but they slaughter hundreds and thousands of rams. Mena is located in a valley, and the pilgrims reside in tents. The majority of pilgrims stay there since the houses are few and very expensive. Unfortunately, the tents are not set up in an orderly fashion and often are set up between the houses. This situation annoys the pilgrims and leads to unhealthy conditions. Thus, the streets should be enlarged and the tents set up in an orderly fashion. The tentmakers should have a map of the places where they should put up their tents. The [campground] should not house more than 1,000 pilgrims and it should be surrounded by a high wall.[64]

He believed that this was an essential task to prevent disease given his claim that there were somewhere between 200,000 and 1 million carcasses to deal with each year at Mena. He recommended that soldiers 'form a cordon between the slaughterhouse and the pilgrims' residences at dawn on the first day of the festival . . . [in order to prevent] the slaughter of rams in the pilgrim's tents. Furthermore, he required that 'the sanitary police and physicians inspect the rams' before they were sold at a secure slaughterhouse, also supervised by sanitary administrative officials.[65]

The locals, however, balked at the measures, as regulating and taxing their trade in sacrificial rams would lessen their income. In 1910, İzzeddin enforced the new rules only because he ordered Fazil Bey Efendi, the son of Hussein, the Sharif of Mecca, 'to send the Bedouins away with their sheep'.[66] The next year he was not so successful:

> It was amazing to see the hostility [of locals] towards Muslim pilgrims and the sanitary services in 1911. Because of this precautions could not be taken against cholera . . . Some [newspapers in Istanbul] condemned the attack . . . [It occurred] after a quarrel between soldiers and Bedouins broke the cordon established by the divisional general Münir Pasha. The Bedouins then brought in herds of sheep to the pilgrims who slaughtered them. We were not able to bury the rams, and this increased the cholera deaths.[67]

CONCLUSION

İzzeddin and the Ottoman sanitary reforms soon went into a fatal tailspin. British mechanical support and supplies of coal – so vital to maintaining Jeddah's and Basra's water and electricity – were effectively cut off after the Ottoman entrance into the First World War on behalf of the Central Powers in November 1914. The railway projects to Baghdad and the Hijaz were incomplete, and sufficient supplies and military reinforcements could not reach the sanitary administration due to the British domination of the Red Sea and Persian Gulf. The local population, once enthusiastic about technological improvements, now had to suffer through depravity. The weakness of Ottoman government was on full display. The British replaced Clemow, their friendly representative to the Ottoman Empire, with the likes of Lieutenant J. T. Lawrence ('Lawrence of Arabia') and other British agents, who stirred animosities between the Ottomans and the disaffected Bedouins.

Sharif Hussein and his sons, once İzzeddin's reluctant agents of reform, now worked with Lawrence to stir up the Bedouins, who themselves were embittered by İzzeddin's treatment of them as a diseased people who could be taxed in the name of centralising sanitary reform.

The Arab Revolt of 1916–18 eventually led to political power for Sharif Hussein's progeny: his sons Faisal and Ali took power in Iraq and the Hijaz, respectively. Now it was their turn to run the sanitary administration. Ironically, they both largely followed in the footsteps of their Ottoman predecessors. In Iraq, Faisal passed the Corpse Traffic Law (1924), which followed earlier

Ottoman controls by severely restricting the pilgrim's import of 'moist corpses'. They were allowed in from outside the country only if they were in 'hermetically sealed . . . coffins lined with iron, lead or zinc to the satisfaction of the inspecting doctor at the town of entry' and had a 'certificate from the foreign authorities or from an Iraqi consular officer . . . that the corpse had not died from an infectious disease'. In addition, the Iraqis only permitted 'moist corpses' to cross the border between 1 November and 31 March.[68]

Ali tried to re-establish the Abu Saad quarantine station and the facilities in Jeddah, Mecca, Medina and Yanbu, but soon felt the brunt of European disdain:

> No effective measures of general sanitation have been taken within the [Hijaz] Kingdom or at the sacred cities, and there is no medical service which in modern eyes could be considered satisfactory. In regard to the ports of the Hijaz, Jeddah and Yanbu, the position is worse than formerly. While the sanitary measures at these ports were undertaken by the Superior Board of Health of Constantinople, they could be applied with due reference to the measures taken in, and information received from, other ports and quarantine stations directed by that board, notably Kamaran. This is not now the case.[69]

He replied in frustration to such reports that he could 'fumigate just as well as the English'.[70] This was a bad sign for Ali's and the Sharif's supporters in the Hijaz. Their Saudi rivals would soon take over the region after Hussein claimed the title of Caliph in 1924.

The Turks faced similar pressures. The British occupied Istanbul after the Ottoman surrender in October 1918. Clemow, who returned with the forces, reported that plague had broken out soon after their arrival:

> In Constantinople plague reappeared, after a long absence, in September, 1919. The source of infection was unknown; but the first cases occurred in connection with the granary. Between September and 19 January 1920, fifty-four cases, with nineteen deaths, were registered. After a plague-free interval the disease broke out again in April, and since 24 April, fifty-six cases have been recorded.[71]

A League of Nations commission sent to study the outbreak highlighted the need for the British to take action:

> Constantinople town and port itself presents special dangers of epidemic diseases which might have a widespread effect in many countries with which it has sea or land communications. The town and all its outlying parts at the present time are overcrowded, and contain a large alien population, most of which is in a state

of destitution and malnutrition. Its internal sanitation and health administration, before the war and until the armistice, were entirely in Turkish hands and generally unsatisfactory. The exceptional conditions which arose in Constantinople after the armistice created a very serious state of affairs as regards public health. Since the Allied occupation a number of emergency measures have been taken under the direction of an international committee, and they have been executed under the supervision of a medical officer of one of the Allied forces. Good results have been obtained in several directions. In regards to epidemics, vigorous action has been taken to deal with plague, which appeared in 1919 and still occurs sporadically, and also with epidemics such as smallpox and typhus. For plague, smallpox and cholera, vaccination or preventative inoculation has been carried out on a very large scale. So far as the limited resources and personnel have permitted, attention has been given to the formidable task of sanitary surveillance of refugees. The whole population, estimated at well over 1 million, however, is still without an infectious diseases hospital, without cleansing stations and baths which can deal with typhus and relapsing fever, and without many other primary sanitary requirements.[72]

These claims that the Ottomans neglected 'sanitary affairs and health administration' contrasted sharply with Clemow's praise just before the war for Dr Cemil Pasha (1858–1968), who was head of the sanitary efforts in Istanbul:

The energetic prefect of the city, Dr Djemil Pasha, is not only enlarging the streets and embellishing the quarters of Istanbul, Pera and Scutari, but he is also doing his best to improve the sanitary and hygienic conditions of our metropolis. The municipal authorities did well to elect for this supervising office a capable and travelled physician with studied Western ways and is in touch with modern ideas. His chief plan for the present is to erect a number of new municipal hospitals worthy of the capital, and to enlarge and improve those already in existence. He has prepared a very extensive report on the matter, and hopes to realise this project in the course of five years.[73]

The League of Nations ignored earlier reports of progress and recommended that the remaining Turkish quarantines be 'internationalised' in much the same way as the Suez Canal and Red Sea quarantine systems had been. This is evident in the following article they drafted for a proposed International Sanitary Conference on the subject:

Measures at Constantinople and the Black Sea Ports: . . . If and when a port sanitary authority having an international character is established at Constantinople,

> such authority shall make regulations of a similar nature to those authorised in the case of the Sanitary Maritime and Quarantine Board of Egypt . . . subject to their acceptance by the powers represented on the authority. The sanitary authority may also take measures in regard to ships from the Black Sea ports which pass through the Bosporus, bound for the Mediterranean, similar to those authorised . . . in the case of ships coming from the south through the Suez Canal and bound for the Mediterranean. In pursuance of these duties this sanitary authority shall provide at a suitable station, or stations, near the northern entrance of the Bosporus, all necessary accommodation for medical examination, disinfection, isolation of sick and observation of contacts.[74]

The Turkish independence movement, led by Mustafa Kemal Atatürk (1881–1938), was in no mood to accept such terms. Turkish nationalist forces entered Istanbul in 1923, signalling the end of any significant British presence in the Straits and Anatolia. The British public may have been sympathetic to local Greeks and the initial occupation of the city, but they were loath to maintain any troop commitments after the long and bloody war. Atatürk and the new Turkish government sensed this weakness, and sent İsmet Inönü, Ataturk's right-hand man, to the Lausanne Peace Conference (1923) to draw up a peace treaty between the new state and the victors of the First World War. Inönü successfully defended Turkey's right to run its own quarantine facilities, and even nationalised the Constantinople Superior Health Council.

The Ottoman Empire's eighty-year experiment in quarantines and sanitary administration had ended with mixed results. The Istanbul quarantine was consistently successful in defending Ottoman interests in the Straits through the government's control of the Constantinople Superior Health Council and the popular support reformers like Hamdan and Ahmed Midhat had garnered. But İzzeddin's sanitary administration's attempt to cement Arab–Turkish ties could not ultimately subjugate the Bedouins of the Hijaz and the Shiites of southern Iraq. Clemow and the British withdrew their support for these efforts after the war broke out and rebellions ensued. Thus, the Ottomans had learned a bitter lesson about quarantine reform: it could help consolidate a republic but not an empire.

NOTES

1. Meclis-i Umur-ı Tıbbiye-i Mülkiye ve Sıhhiye-i Umumiye, *Veba*, p. 24.
2. Meclis-i Umur-ı Tıbbiye-i Mülkiye ve Sıhhiye-i Umumiye, *Veba*, pp. 7–8.
3. Dr F. G. Clemow, 'Cholera, the Haj, and the Hedjaz Railway', *The Lancet* 20 February 1909, pp. 577–78.
4. Ministére des affaires étrangères, *Conférence Sanitaire Internatiionale de Paris: 7 Novembre 1911–17 Janvier 1912: Procès-verbaux*, pp. 432, 434.

5. Ruhi Al-Khailidi's relative Nazif Bey al-Khalidi (1875–1916) was a key engineer for the Hijaz Railway, helping to construct the main railway terminal in Damascus and lines in what is now modern-day Syria and Jordan. William Ochsenwald, *The Hijaz Railway*, p. 34. See also see: Hasan Kayalı, 'Arabs and Young Turks: Ottomanism, Arabism, and Islamism in the Ottoman Empire, 1908–1918', pp. 104–5.
6. Dr Bartoletti, *Rapport sur les Measures à Prendre Contre la Peste Qui Sévit en Perse*, pp. 3–11.
7. Tholozan, *Histoire de la Peste Bubonique*, pp. 1–42.
8. Simpson, *A Treatise on Plague*, p. 436.
9. Dr F. G. Clemow, 'The Shiah Pilgrimage and the Sanitary Defences of Mesopotamia and the Turco-Persian Frontier', *The Lancet* 12 August 1916, p. 290.
10. Clemow, 'Shiah Pilgrimage', 2 September 1916, p. 442.
11. Clemow, 'Shiah Pilgrimage', 19 August 1916, p. 334.
12. Clemow, 'Shiah Pilgrimage', 19 August 1916, p. 334.
13. Clemow, 'Shiah Pilgrimage', 9 September 1916, p. 490.
14. Clemow, 'Shiah Pilgrimage', 2 September 1916, pp. 442–3.
15. Clemow, 'Shiah Pilgrimage', 9 September 1916, pp. 490–1
16. Clemow, 'Shiah Pilgrimage', 12 August 1916, p. 293; 2 September 1916, p. 442.
17. Clemow, 'Shiah Pilgrimage', 12 August 1916, p. 290.
18. Clemow, 'Shiah Pilgrimage', 2 September 1916, p. 442; 12 August 1916, p. 290.
19. Clemow, 'Shiah Pilgrimage', 9 September 1916, p. 490.
20. Cassim İzzeddine, *Le Pèlerinage Chiite et l'Hygiène*, pp. 43–61.
21. İzzeddine, *Le Pèlerinage*, p. 6.
22. Clemow, 'Shiah Pilgrimage', 12 August 1916, p. 290.
23. Lamec Saad, *Sechsen Jahre als Quarantänearzt in der Türkei*, p. 63. I want to thank Dr York Norman for translating the relevant passages from this text from German to English.
24. Ministére des affaires étrangères, *Conférence Sanitaire Internatiionale*, p. 801.
25. Ministére des affaires étrangères, *Conférence Sanitaire Internatiionale*, p. 797.
26. Dr F. G. Clemow, 'The Sanitary Defence of the Hedjaz Railway', *The Lancet* 24 October 1908, p. 1250.
27. Clemow, 'The Sanitary Defence of the Hedjaz Railway', 7 November 1908, p. 1406.
28. Clemow, 'The Sanitary Defence of the Hedjaz Railway', 10 October 1908, p. 1104.
29. Ochsenwald, *Hijaz Railway*, pp. 138–9.
30. Ministére des affaires étrangères, *Conférence Sanitaire Internatiionale*, p. 270.
31. Proust, *La Défense de Europe*, pp. 242–3.
32. İzzeddin, *Hicaz'da Teşkilat (1329)*, pp. 11–12.
33. Michael C. Low, 'Empire of the Hajj: Pilgrims, Plagues and Pan-Islam under British Surveillance, 1865–1926', pp. 102–3.
34. Proust, *La Défense de Europe*, p. 243.
35. İzzeddin, *Hicaz'da Teşkilat (1329)*, pp. 64–7.
36. The Hijaz Railway had an annual budget of ranging between 1,033,465 paistres (1903) and 3,975,443 paistres (1908). Ochsenwald, *Hijaz Railway*, p. 80.
37. İzzeddin, *Hicaz'da Teşkilat (1329)*, pp. 13, 36, 47–9.
38. İzzeddin, *Hicaz'da Teşkilat (1329)*, pp. 47–9.
39. İzzeddin, *Hicaz'da Teşkilat (1330)*, pp. 3, 27–8, 64, 76–81; Kayalı, 'Arabs and Young Turks', pp. 165–8.

40. Dr F. G. Clemow, 'Some Turkish Lazarets and Other Sanitary Institutions in the Near East', *The Lancet* 29 June 1907, p. 1811.
41. İzzeddin, *Hicaz'da Teşkilat (1329)*, p. 40.
42. İzzeddin, *Hicaz'da Teşkilat (1329)*, pp. 76–81.
43. Low, 'Empire of the Hajj', pp 102–3.
44. Clemow, 'Turkish Lazarets', 29 June 1907, pp. 1811–12; 6 July 1907, pp. 51–2; F. G. Clemow, *Le Eaux de Djeddah*, pp. 3–7.
45. Clemow, *Le Eaux de Djeddah*, p. 7.
46. Clemow, 'Turkish Lazarets', 6 July 1907, p. 52.
47. Clemow, 'Turkish Lazarets', 6 July 1907, p. 52.
48. İzzeddin, *Hicaz'da Teşkilat (1330)*, pp. 76–81.
49. İzzeddin, *Hicaz'da Teşkilat (1330)*, p. 42.
50. İzzeddin, *Hicaz'da Teşkilat (1330)*, p. 51.
51. Ochsenwald, *Hijaz Railway*, p. 99.
52. Donald Quataert, *The Ottoman Empire, 1700–1922*, front cover.
53. İzzeddin, *Hicaz'da Teşkilat (1330)*, pp. 51, 61.
54. İzzeddin, *Hicaz'da Teşkilat (1330)*, p. 61.
55. İzzeddin, *Hicaz'da Teşkilat (1330)*, p. 64.
56. York Norman, 'Are Muslims "Jews" or "Gypsies"? A Reassessment of Bosnian Muslim Political Thought under the Habsburgs', p. 4. I thank Dr Norman for letting me read his unpublished work.
57. İzzeddin, *Hicaz'da Teşkilat (1330)*, pp. 54, 56.
58. Dr F. G. Clemow, 'Egypt', *The Lancet* 10 March 1906, p. 718.
59. İzzeddin, *Hicaz'da Teşkilat (1330)*, 56.
60. İzzeddin, *Hicaz'da Teşkilat (1330)*, pp. 24–5, 60–1.
61. İzzeddin, *Hicaz'da Teşkilat (1330)*, pp. 24–5.
62. Clemow, 'Turkish Lazarets', 4 May 1907, p. 1253.
63. Clemow, 'Turkish Lazarets', 4 May 1907, p. 1253.
64. İzzeddin, *Hicaz'da Teşkilat (1329)*, 45–6.
65. İzzeddin, *Hicaz'da Teşkilat (1330)*, 24–5.
66. İzzeddin, *Hicaz'da Teşkilat (1329)*, pp. 78–9.
67. İzzeddin, *Hicaz'da Teşkilat (1330)*, p. 137.
68. Anja Pistor-Hatam, 'Pest und Cholera: Die Wahlfahrt zu den Heilegen Stätten im Irak als gesundheitspolitisches Problem im 19. Jahrhundert', pp. 243–4.
69. League of Nations, *Report of Commission*, 20 February–27 March 1922, p. 8.
70. Sean Foley, *The Arab Gulf States: Beyond Oil and Islam*, p. 215.
71. Dr F. G. Clemow, 'Plague in Turkey during the War', *The Lancet* 20 November 1920, p. 1065.
72. League of Nations, *Report of Commission*, 20 February–27 March 1922, pp. 11–12.
73. Dr F. G. Clemow, 'Constantinople', *The Lancet* 28 March 1914, p. 927.
74. League of Nations, *Report of Commission*, 20 February–27 March 1922, pp. 22–3.

CHAPTER

8

TOWARDS A NEW UNDERSTANDING OF PLAGUE AND QUARANTINES IN THE OTTOMAN EMPIRE

This book argues that Hamdan Bin El-Merhum Osman Hoca was indeed a pivotal figure in the history of plague in the Ottoman Empire, as his vision of quarantine as an instrument of national sovereignty had the most lasting political impact on the Ottoman medical reforms about epidemic disease.

Before his time the Ottomans had an essentially premodern view of plague and other epidemic diseases. Although the Ottomans traditionally conceived of plague and health in ways that that did not contradict their ruling Islamic faith, they reacted to the Black Death and later outbreaks of plague much in the same way as their medieval European counterparts. Many of their most prominent writers (Al-Yahudi, Bitlisi and Taşköprüzade) generally thought that plague began with a miasmatic corruption of the air that killed humans and animals alike by causing a fatal elemental imbalance. They prescribed cures and methods of fumigation that were virtually identical to that of their northern neighbours. Some even shared Boccaccio's and Fracastoro's belief that the plague was spread by contagion. Yet only Venice and a small number of Italian city-states used the idea of contagion to justify the building of maritime quarantines in the late fourteenth and fifteenth centuries. Still, almost all plague treatise writers, Ottomans and Europeans included, believed that their readers should undertake whatever medical, spiritual and magical precautions and cures they could to combat the disease. The writers most often felt their task was to add to their knowledge, regardless of whether it was medical or not.

This pattern changed when the European maritime powers began their commercial and colonial overseas expansion. The British, the most successful of these powers, were instrumental in the further development of quarantine practices. They used the idea of contagion to justify banning textiles and peoples from 'suspected' countries – often a convenient policy for English entrepreneurs, who wished to sell domestic textiles instead of that of their Dutch and French rivals. Contagionist beliefs also often legitimised greater controls against the poor, minorities and immigrants from abroad. Controversies about the policies often had a political tinge that reflected social, religious and colonial divides among the body politic. Debates about these measures were discussed in an emerging press culture that transformed both author and audience. The author – who previously wrote for small, courtly circles of patrons – now had to tailor his message to meet the needs of a large, commercial elite. As a result, English plague treatises revolved much more around commerce and quarantine policy than they did about previously popular magical or spiritual 'cures' for the plague. Those who persisted faced likely persecution as religious dissidents or even witches.

The Ottomans began to change their views of plague and quarantine in the decades after Napoleon's invasion of Egypt in 1798. It was only after this first attempt by Europeans to colonise the Middle East that the Ottomans realised that they would have to adopt quarantine as part of a greater modernisation project. Hamdan, the medical architect of the reforms, saw this threat first-hand when the French invaded his native Algeria in 1830. He supported the adoption of an Ottoman maritime quarantine system as a mercantilist tool to resist outside intervention in the Empire's commercial, social and political affairs. He also called for the quarantine and other public health issues to be discussed in print.[1] This wish became reality after Hamdan wrote his treatise, as an emerging Ottoman press published works on plague from that time onwards.

Importantly, Hamdan refused to accept the social disciplinary aspects of quarantine reform. He did not blame the poor, religious minorities or ethnic groups for spreading plague. These views might only be partially explained by Hamdan's abhorrence for colonialism and the European medical institutions that helped to rationalise them. They also fitted fully within the general Ottoman philosophy to adopt only those parts of modernising reform that could be reconciled with their governing philosophy and faith. Hamdan's successors would not implement major medical policing measures within the Empire until the Paris International Sanitary Conference in 1894, when they were pressured to do so by the European powers.

The British and French reacted to Hamdan by revising their notions of plague. They supported a seminal 1846 study of plague in Egypt by Clot-Bey and Aubert-Roche, which posited that plague was infectious, spread by poor hygiene and environmental factors rather than contagiously spread by human to human contact. They found that only unclean and undeveloped countries were endemic with the disease. In their eyes, European 'civilised nations' should not fear plague spreading to them through international travel and trade. The Europeans supposedly combated the disease abroad by promoting public health and other sanitary improvements in the underdeveloped world. These conclusions validated further English and French commercial penetration of the Middle East, the colonisation of Egypt and the construction of the Suez Canal.

The establishment of a new infectionist-based medical inspection quarantine system at the Suez Canal and the Red Sea was an even greater humiliation for the Ottomans than the internationalisation of the Constantinople Superior Health Council in 1838. The Ottomans still dominated the Council and its affiliated quarantines in Istanbul, the Black Sea and much of the eastern Mediterranean, but they began to lose control of their Arab provinces, particularly the Hijaz.

The Ottomans reacted by adopting infectionism, especially the idea of medically policing the social and religious marginal groups of the Empire. Kasım İzzeddin, the head of Ottoman sanitation efforts in Iraq and the Hijaz from 1894 to 1912, hoped to consolidate the Arab provinces of the Empire by targeting the poor, the Bedouins and the Shiites as risk groups for plague and other epidemic diseases. İzzeddin, a Lebanese Arab, provides interesting contrasts with Hamdan, the earlier Ottoman reformer, who also came from the Arab frontiers of the Empire. Both inaugurated their reforms in the hope of avoiding impending colonisation, but their policies were strikingly different. Whereas Hamdan successfully convinced a sceptical domestic audience to support the quarantine, İzzeddin gained international support – especially from the British – but embittered the Hijaz Bedouins and Iraqi Shiites in the process. Hamdan rejected sanitary policing measures as colonialist, but İzzeddin tried to use medical inspection along with new technologies (railways, urban improvements, water distilling and ice machines) to consolidate the empire.

The British were key to İzzeddin's success as they provided the coal, water distilling and ice machines, and much-needed transportation. Yet the outbreak of war in 1914, when the Ottoman Empire joined the Central powers against Britain and her allies, effectively doomed İzzeddin's project. The British ended their shipments of coal and supply, started shelling the Hijaz ports, and provoked rebellion among the Bedouins. Hussein, the Sharif of Mecca and leader of the Hijaz Bedouins, no doubt felt that İzzeddin's medical inspections, sanitation and technological developments were part of the greater Ottoman attempt to 'colonise' the Arabian Peninsula.

Only the Ottoman quarantine in Istanbul would emerge intact from the First World War. The British would temporarily take over the quarantine facilities and administrative headquarters on the Golden Horn, but this bred resentment among the Turks – now themselves a marginal group who wished to reassert their sovereignty. When Inönü – Atatürk's plenipotentiary at the Lausanne Peace Conference – won the concession that the Republic of Turkey would control the quarantine, Hamdan's dream had come true at last.

NOTE

1. Hamdan, *Tercüme-i İthaf*, fol. 35A.

BIBLIOGRAPHY

PRIMARY SOURCES

Abdullah, Derviş, *Müfredat*, Ghazi Husrev Beg Library, R-2461, 1737.

Abdullah, Yusuf Ali, *The Meaning of the Holy Quran*, New edition, revised translation, commentary and newly compiled comprehensive index (Beltsville, MD: Amana Publications, 1997).

Ahmed bin Halil er-Rumi, İshak Hocası, *Risale fi İlmi Tılsım ve Def'i''t-Taun*, Süleymaniye Library, Pertev Paşa 618, 1708.

Al-Ghazali, Ebu Hamid Muhammed b. Muhammed, *Cünnetü'l-Esmai'l-Mücerrebe li'l Vebai ve't-Taun*, Hacı Selimağa Library, Kemankeş 303 (undated).

Al-Yahudi, İlyas bin Abram, *Micennetü't-Ta'un ve'l-Veba*, trans. Kürkzade Hafız Hasan, İstanbul Merkez Kütüphanesi, No. 1299, 1801.

Anonymous, *The Graces Folowying be Graunted* . . . 1520.

Anonymous, *The Mourning Cross, or Lord Have Mercy Upon Us* . . . (London, 1665).

Anonymous, *The Plague as It Affects England from Official and Other Sources* (London: Hardwick and Bogue, 1879).

Anonymous, *Church of Englandman's Companion*, 1731.

Anonymous, *Church of England*, 1756.

Arnaud, Dr L. *Essai sur la Peste de Benghazi en 1874: Rapport Addresé au Conseil Supérioir de Santé de Constantinople* (Constantinople: Typographie et Lithographie Centrales, 1875).

Balmford, James, *A Short Dialogue concerning the Plague's Infection published to preserue Bloud, through the Blessing of God: Together with a Sorting of all those Verses in the Psalmes which are noted with the Word Selah to shew the Complaints, Comforts, Faith, Prayer and Praise of God's Children* (London: Printed by W. Iones, 1625), pp. 22–4.

Barker, Christopher, *England and Wales Sovereign by the Queene: A Proclamation against the Bringing in of Wines from Bordeaux in Respect to Plague being there* . . . (London, ca 1592).

Bartoletti, Dr, 'La Peste de Benghazi', *La Gazzette Medicale d'Orient II* (1858–9): 105–11.

Bartoletti, Dr, *Rapport sur les Measures à Prendre Contre la Peste Qui Sévit en Perse* (Constantinople: Typographie et Lithographie Centrales, 1871).

Bartoletti, Dr, *Rapport sur la Perception de la Taxe Sanitaire Statistique de la Navigation dans les Ports Ottomans du 1er Mars au 28 Février 1879 et Bilan de Recette et de la Dépense du Service Pendant la Même Année Présenté au Conseil Supérioir de Santé* (Constantinople: Typographie et Lithographie Centrales, 1880).

Bašeski, Molla Mustafa Ševki, *Ljetopis, 1749–1804*, trans. Mehmed Mujezinović (Sarajevo: Veselin Masleša, 1968).

Beza, Théodore de Bèze, *A Learned Treatise of the Plague Wherein the Two Questions, Whether the Plague be Infectious or No, and, Whether and How Farr it May be Shunned of Christians by Going Aside, Are Resolved* (London: Printed by Thomas Ratcliffe, 1580).

Bitlisi, İdris-i, *Hısn ül-veba: Terceme-i risalet ül-veba*, trans. Muhammed Salih, Süleymaniye Library, Hacı Mahmud Efendi 4015, 1827.

Boccaccio, Giovanni, *The Decameron*, trans. Guido Waldman (Oxford: Oxford University Press, 1993).

Brooks, Thomas, *A Heavenly Cordial for all those Servants of the Lord that have had the Plague . . . , or, Thirteen Divine Maximes, or Conclusions, in Respect of the Pestilence: Which may be as so Many Supports, Comforts and Refreshing Springs, both to the Visited and Preserved People of God in this Present Day: Also Ten Arguments to Prove that in Times of Common Calamity the People of God do stand upon the Advantage Ground as to their Outward Preservation and Protection . . .: Also Eight Reasons why some of the Precious Servants of the Lord have fallen by the Pestilence in this Day of the Lord's Anger* (London: Printed for and to be sold by John Hancock, 1666).

Clarke, Samuel, *Sermons on Several Subjects and Occasions by Samuel Clarke, . . . In Eight Volumes. Containing One-Hundred and Ninety-One Discourses, Being all those Published in his Life-Time, and those Since his Death, by John Clarke, . . . With a Preface, . . . by Benjamin, Now Lord Bishop of Winchester* (London: Printed for A. Millar, J. and R. Tonson, J. Hodges, W. Bowyer, R. Baldwin, S. Crowder and H. Woodgate, 1756).

Clemow, Dr F. G., *Le Eaux de Djeddah* (Constantinople: Impremerie F. Loeffler, Lithographe de S. M. I. le Sultan, 1906).

Clemow, Dr F. G., 'Constantinople', *The Lancet* 6 January 1906, pp. 64–5; 20 January 1906, pp. 192–3; 14 April 1906, pp. 1082–3; 9 June 1906, p. 1647; 23 June 1906, p. 1795; 27 July 1912, p. 265; 23 November 1912; pp. 1470–1; 28 March 1914, p. 927.

Clemow, Dr F. G., 'Egypt', *The Lancet* 10 March 1906, p. 718.

Clemow, Dr F. G., 'Some Turkish Lazarets and Other Sanitary Institutions in the Near East', *The Lancet* 27 April 1907, pp. 1188–9; 4 May 1907, pp. 1251–3; 18 May 1907, pp. 1389–92; 11 May 1907, pp. 1317–20; 1 June 1907, pp. 1518–21; 8 June 1907, pp. 1607–10; 22 June 1907, pp. 1741–3; 29 June 1907, pp. 1810–12; 6 July 1907, pp. 51–2; 13 July 1907, pp. 114–18; 20 July 1907, pp. 190–2; 3 August 1907, pp. 324–5.

Clemow Dr F. G., 'Cholera in the Pilgrimage and Elsewhere', *The Lancet* 29 February 1908, pp. 678–9.

Clemow, Dr F. G., 'The Sanitary Defence of the Hedjaz Railway', *The Lancet* 25 September 1908.

Clemow, Dr F. G., 'Cholera and Plague in Russia and the Near East', *The Lancet*, 16 January 1909, p. 196; 4 May 1912, pp. 1234–5; 22 June 1912, pp. 1720–1; 17 August 1912, pp. 482–4; 28 September 1912, pp. 912–3; 14 June 1913, pp. 1697–8.

Clemow Dr F. G., 'Cholera and War and the Near East', *The Lancet* 15 February 1913, pp. 484–5.

Clemow, Dr F. G., 'Cholera in the Near East', *The Lancet* 7 February 1914, pp. 406–7; 1 August 1914, pp. 337–8.

Clemow, Dr F. G., 'War and the Danger from Cholera in the Near East', *The Lancet* 10 October 1914, pp. 911–13.

Clemow, Dr. F. G., 'The Shiah Pilgrimage and the Sanitary Defences of Mesopotamia and the Turco-Persian Frontier', *The Lancet* 12 August 1916, pp. 289–93; 19 August 1916, pp. 333–5; 2 September 1916, pp. 441–3; 9 September 1916, pp. 488–91.

Clemow, Dr F. G., 'Plague in Turkey during the War', *The Lancet* 20 November 1920, p. 1065.

Davies, E., *A Sermon Preach'd on Friday Decemb. 16th 1720 being the Day of Publick Fasting and Humiliation for the Averting God's Judgements, particularly the Plague* (London: Printed for T. Hurt, 1721).

Defoe, Daniel, *The Case Fairly Stated between the Turkey Company and the Italian Merchants* (London: Printed by J. Roberts, 1720).

Defoe, Daniel, *The History of the Great Plague in London, in the Year 1665 . . . By a Citizen, who lived the Whole Time in London. To which is added, a Journal of the Plague at Marseilles, in the Year 1720* (London: Printed for and sold by F. and J. Noble, 1754).

Ebussuud Efendi, *Risale-i Ebussuud*, Süleymaniye Library, Denizli No. 43, 1580.

Ellsworth DeKay, James, *Sketches of Turkey in 1831 and 1832* (New York: J. and J. Harper, 1833).

Ertuğrul Düzdağ, Mehmet, *Şeyhülislam Ebussuud Efendi Fetvaları Işığında 16. Asır Türk Hayatı* (İstanbul: Enderun Kitabevi, 1972).

Explainer, *Distinct Notions of the Plague, with the Rise and Fall of Pestilential Contagion. By the Explainer* (London, 1722).

Fracastoro, Girolamo, *De Contagione et Contagiosis Morbis et Eorum Curatione, Libri III* (New York: G. P. Putnam, 1930).

Gadbury, John, *London's Deliverance Predicted in a Short Discourse Shewing the Cause of Plagues in General, and the Probable Time (God Not Contradicting the Course of Second Causes) When the Present Pest May Abate, &c* (London: Printed by J. C., 1665).

Gadbury, John, *Vox Solis: or, an Astrological Discourse of the Great Eclipse of the Sun, which happened on June 22. 1666: in 10 Deg. of the Watry Signe Cancer. Shewing what Effects may most probably attend it, and unto what Persons, Kingdoms and Countries, they are chiefly directed* (London: Printed by James Cotterel, 1667).

Gaffarel, Jacques, *Unheard-of Curiosities: Concerning the Talismanical Sculpture of the Persians; The Horoscope of the Patriarkes; and the Reading of the Stars. Written in French, by James Gaffarel. And Englished by Edmund Chilmead, Mr. of Arts, and Chaplaine of Christ-Church Oxon* (London: Printed by G. D. for Humphrey Moseley, 1650).

Gibbon, Edmond, ed. D. M. Low, *The Decline and Fall of the Roman Empire* (New York: Harcourt, Brace, 1960).

Goldwin, William, *God's Judgments on a Sinful People. A Sermon preach'd on the 8th of December, being the Fast-Day, appointed to implore God's Protection against the Plague now in France* (Bristol: Printed by and for Joseph Penn, 1722).

Graunt, John, *Natural and Political Observations mentioned in a following Index, and made upon the Bills of Mortality* (London: John Martyn and James Allestry, 1665).

Grosvenor, Benjamin, *Preparation for Death, the Best Preservative against the Plague. Being the Substance of Two Sermons, preach'd at the Merchant's Lecture in Salters-Hall, Jan. seventeenth, and 31st, 1721* (London: Printed for John Clark, 1721).

Hamdan Bin Al-Merhum Osman Hoca, *Tercüme-i İthaf el-Munassıfın ve'l-Üdeba bi Mabahit el-İhtiraz'an el-Veba*, Süleymaniye Library: Nafız Paşa 836, 1836.

Hamdan Khodja, *Le Miroir: Aperçu Historique et Statistique sur la Régence d'Alger*, introduction d'Abdelkader Djeghloul (Paris: Sindbad, 1985).

Hastler, Thomas, *An Antidote against the Plague. Or Panchrestōn: A Salve for All Sores: which applied and practised, will soone awaken the Lord's Mercy, and suddenly cause the Storms of his Just Judgements to vanish away. Delivered in a Sermon, preached within the Cathedrall Church of Saint Paules, London* (London: Printed by M. Flesher, 1615).

Hobbes, Thomas, *Leviathan* (Cambridge: Cambridge University Press, 1996).

Hodges, Nathaniel, *Loimologia: or, an Historical Account of the Plague in London in 1665: With Precautionary Directions against the Like Contagion. By Nath. Hodges, M.D. . . . To which is added, An essay on the different causes of pestilential diseases, . . . By John Quincy, M.D.* (London: Printed for E. Bell and J. Osborn, 1721).

Holland, Henry, *Spirituall Preseruatiues against the Pestilence: Or a Treatise containing Sundrie Questions: Both Concerning the Causes of the Pestilence, (Where is Shewed, that the Plague is a Mixt Euill of Knowne and Secret Causes, and therefore so Hardly Healed by Naturall Curatiues only) and the Most Pretious Preseruatiues against the Same and Many Other Euils. Chiefely Collected out of the 91 Psalme.* (London: Printed by R. Field and T. Scarlet, 1593).

Howard, John, *An Account of the Principal Lazarettos in Europe; with Various Papers Relative to the Plague* (Warrington, 1789).

Hughes, Obadiah, *The Good Man's Security in Times of Publick Calamity. A Sermon preach'd in Maid-Lane, Southwark, on Occasion of the Plague in France* (London: Printed for John Clark and John Morley, 1722).

Hull, Charles Henry (ed.), *The Economic Writings of Sir William Petty: Together with the Observations upon the Bills of Mortality more probably by John Graunt* (Fairfield, NJ: A. M. Kelley, 1986).

Hurgonje, C. Snouck, *Mekka in the Latter Part of the Nineteenth Century: The Daily Life, Customs and Learning of the Moslims of the East Indian-Archipelago* (Leiden: E. J. Brill, 1970).

International Sanitary Conference, *Conférence sanitaire internationale de Paris (7 Février–3 Avril 1894): Procès-verbaux* (Paris: Imprimerie nationale, 1894).

International Sanitary Conference, *Procès-verbaux de la Conférence sanitaire internationale ouverte en Paris le 27 Juillet 1851* (Paris: Imprimerie nationale, 1852).

International Sanitary Conference, *Procès-verbaux de la Conférence sanitaire internationale ouverte en a Vienne le 1 Juillet 1874* (Vienne: Imprimerie impériale, 1874).

International Sanitary Conference, *Report to the International Sanitary Conference from a Commission from that Body to which were Referred Questions Relative to the Origin, Transmissibility and Propagation of Asiatic Cholera*, trans. Samuel Abbot (Boston, MA: Alfred Mudge, 1867).

İzzeddine, Cassim, *La défense sanitaire dans le Golfe Persique* (Paris: A. Maloine, 1912).

İzzeddine, Cassim, *Le choléra et l'hygiène à la Mecque* (Paris: A. Maloine, 1909).

İzzeddine, Cassim, *Le pèlerinage Chiite et l'hygiène* (Paris: A. Maloine, 1912).

İzzeddine, Cassim, *Les épidemies de choléra au Hedjaz* (Constantinople: Imprimerie Amiré, 1918).

İzzeddin, Kasım, *Hicaz'da Teşkilat ve Islahat-ı Sıhhiye ve 1329 Senesi Hacc-ı Şerifi, Hicaz Sıhhiye İdaresi, Senevi Raporu* (İstanbul: Matbaa-ı Amire, 1300 [1911 or 1912]).

İzzeddin, Kasım, *Hicaz'da Teşkilat ve Islahat-ı Sıhhiye ve 1330 Senesi Hacc-ı Şerifi, Hicaz Sıhhiye İdaresi, Senevi Raporu* (İstanbul: Matbaa-ı Amire, 1330 [1911 or 1912]).

Jabarti, Abd al-Rahmān, *Napoleon in Egypt: Al-Jabartī's Chronicle of the French Occupation, 1798*, Introduction Robert L. Tignor, trans. Shmuel Moreh (Princeton, NJ: Markus Wiener, 2004).

Kellwaye, Simon, *A Defensatiue against the Plague: Contayning Two Partes or Treatises: The First, Shewing the Meanes How to Preserue Us from the Dangerous Contagion thereof: The Second, How to Cure Those that are Infected Therewith. Whereunto is annexed a Short Treatise of the Small Poxe: Shewing how to Gouerne and Helpe Those that are Infected therewith* (London: Iohn Windet, 1593).

Kemp, William, *A Brief Treatise of the Nature, Causes, Signes, Preservation from, and Cure of the Pestilence* (London: Printed for D. Kemp, 1665).

Lago, Anton, *Risale-i Karantina*, Süleymaniye Library: Esad Efendi 2482, 1836.

League of Nations, *Report of Commission to Inquire into International Arrangements regarding Epidemic Disease Prevention in Certain Areas of the Near East (Basin of the Eastern Mediterranean and Black Sea) and in Connection with the Mecca Pilgrimage*, 20 February–27 March 1922, With Annex Modification Proposed in Parts Two and Three of the International Sanitary Convention, 1912. Presented to the Health Committee 11 May 1922 (Boston, MA: World Peace Foundation, 1922).

Lilly, William, *England's Propheticall Merline, foretelling to all Nations of Europe untill 1663. The Actions depending upon the Influence of the Conjunction of Saturn and Jupiter, 1642/3. The Progresse and Motion of the Comet 1618. Under Whole Effects we in England, and Most Regions of Europe now suffer. What Kingdomes must yet partake of the Remainder of the Influence, viz. of War, Plague, Famine, etc. When the English Commonwealth may expect Peace, and the City of London Better Times. The Beginning, and End of the Watry Trygon: An Entrance of the Fiery Triplicity, 1603. The Nativities of some English Kings, and some Horary Question inserted: performed by William Lilly, Student in Astrologie* (London: Printed by John Raworth for John Partridge, 1644).

Machiavelli, Niccolo, *The Prince*, ed. James B. Atkinson (Indianapolis, IN: Bobbs-Merrill, 1976).

Maclean, Charles, *Results of an Investigation Respecting Epidemic and Pestilential Diseases; including Researches in the Levant concerning the Plague* (London: Thomas and George Underwood, 1818).

Mead, Richard, *A Short Discourse concerning Pestilential Contagion, or the Plague, with the Methods to be used to prevent it* (Cork, 1721).

Mead, Richard, *A Discourse on the Plague: by Richard Mead . . .* (London: Printed for A. Millar and J. Brindley, 1744).

Meclis-i Umur-ı Tıbbiye-i Mülkiye ve Sıhhiye-i Umumiye, *Veba* (İstanbul: Tanin Matbaası, 1908).

Metzger, Bruce, *et al.*, *The New Oxford Annotated Bible with the Apocrypha: An Ecumenical Study Bible Completely Revised and Enlarged* (New York: Oxford University Press, 1991).

Midhat, Ahmed, 'Devlet-i aliyye-i Osmâniye'de Karantina Yani Usûl-I Tahaffuzun Târihçesi', trans. Abdullah Köşe, *Osmanlı Bilimi Araştırmaları* 5(1) (2003): 89–119.

Milroy, Gavin, *Quarantine and the Plague: Being a Summary of a Report on these Subjects Recently Addressed to the Academy of Medicine in France: With Introductory Observations, Extracts from Parliamentary Correspondence and Notes* (London: Samuel Highley, 1846).

Ministère des affaires étrangères, *Conférence sanitaire internationale de Paris: 7 Novembre 1911–17 Janvier 1912: Procès-verbaux* (Paris: Impremerie nationale, 1912).

Montagu, Lady Mary Wortley, *Turkish Embassy Letters*, eds Anita Desai and Malcolm Jack (Athens, GA: University of Georgia, 1993).

Morgan, Thomas, *A Common Prayer-Book, according to the Plan of the Liturgy of the Church of England, with Suitable Services* (Exeter: Printed by T. Brice, 1791).

Mordtmann, Bartoletti and Stécoulis, Drs, *Le Pèlerinage de 1883 et la Quarantine de Camaran: Rapport au Conseil Supérior de Santé* (Constantinople: Typographie et Lithographie du Journal 'La Turquie', 1883).

Moulton, Thomas, *This is the Myrrour or Glasse of Helth Necessary and Nedefull for Euery Person to Loke in, That wil Kepe their Bodye from the Syckenesse of the Pestilence, and it Sheweth howe the Planettes do Raygne in euery Houre of the Daye and Nyghte, with the Natures and Exposicio[n]s of the xii Sygnes, Deuyded by the. xii. Monethes of the Yeare, and shewed the Remedies for many dyuers Infirmities and Dyseases that hurteth the Bodye of Mann* (London: T. Colwell, 1561).

Muhiddin, Dr, *Sıhhat ve Hayat-ı İslam* (İstanbul: Dersaadet, Mahmud Bey Matbaası, 1907).

Müstakimzade, Sa'deddin Süleyman bin Muhammed Emin, *Cihazü'l-Macun fi'l-Halas Mine't-Taun*, Süleymaniye Library: Esad Efendi: 1329, 1780.

Newton, Benjamin, *Sermons on Several Occasions. In Two Volumes* (London: A. Bettesworth and C. Hitch, 1736).

Noyan, Abdülkadir, *Son Harplerde Salgın Hastalıklarla Savaşlarım* (Ankara: Son Havadis Matbaası, 1956).

Oldenburg, Henry, *The Correspondence of Henry Oldenburg, vol. 2: 1663–1665*, eds and trans. A. Rupert Hall and Marie Boas Hall (Madison, WI: University of Wisconsin Press, 1966).

Ömer Besim, 'Veba-Ta'un', *Servet-i Fünun* 19 (1898): 218–21, 226–37.

Penah, Osman bin Süleyman, *Risale-i Taun*. Süleymaniye Library: Serez 2920, 1804.

Porter, Sir James, *Observations on the Religion, Law, Government, and Manners of the Turks. The Second Edition, Corrected and Enlarged by the Author. To which is . . .* (London, 1771).

Proust, Adrien, *La défense de Europe contre la peste et la Conférence de Venise de 1897* (Paris: Masson et Cie, 1897).

Rifat Paşa, İbrahim, *Mir'atü'l Harameyn bir Generalin Hac Notları*, trans. Lütfüllah Yavuz (İstanbul: Yitik Hazine Yayınları, 2010).

Russell, Alexander, *Natural History of Aleppo, 1742–1744*, vol. 2. (London, 1756).

Russell, Patrick, *A Treatise of the Plague: Containing an Historical Journal, and Medical Account, of the Plague, at Aleppo, in the years 1760, 1761, and 1762 . . .* (London, 1791).

Saad, Lamec, *Sechsen Jahre als Quarantänearzt in der Türkei* (Berlin: Dietrich Reimer, 1913).

Simpson, William J., *A Treatise on Plague dealing with the Historical, Epidemiological, Clinical, Therapeutic and Preventative Aspects of the Disease* (London: Cambridge University Press, 1905).

Smith, Adam, *The Wealth of Nations* (New York: Collier & Son, 1909).

Süreyyā, Mehmed, *Sicill-i Osmanī* (İstanbul: Tarih Vakfı Yurt Yayınları, 1996).

Süreyyā, Mehmed, *Sicill-i Osmanī, İstanbul, 1308/1890–1315/1897* (Westmead: Gregg International Publishers, 1971).

Tahsin, Rıza, *Mirat-i Mekteb-i Tibbiye* (İstanbul: Dersaadet Kadir Matbaası, 1910).

Taşköprüzade, Kemaleddin, *Risale fi't-Taun ve'l-Veba*, trans. Abdulgani Efendi, Süleymaniye Library, Aşir Efendi 275, 1586.

Tholozan, Joseph-Désiré, *Histoire de la Peste Bubonique en Perse ou Détermination de la Son Origine de la Marche, du Cycle, de ses Apparitions et de la Cause de sa Prompte Extinction* (Paris: Libraire l'académie de médcine, 1874).

Tholozan, Joseph-Désiré, *La Peste en Turquie dans les Temps Moderns: Sa Prophylaxie Défectueuse, sa Limitation Spontanée* (Paris: Masson, 1880).

Thucydides, *The History of the Peloponnesian War, by Thucydides. A New and Literal Version, from the Text of Arnold, Collated with Bekker, Göller, and Poppo. By the Rev. Henry Dale* (London: Bell and Daldy, 1872–5).

Urquhart, David, *Turkey and its Resources: Its Municipal Organization and Free Trade; the State and Prospects of English Commerce in the East, the New Administration of Greece, its Revenue and National Possessions* (London: Saunders and Otley, 1833).

Wavell, A. J. B., *A Modern Pilgrim in Mecca and a Siege in Sanaa* (London: Constable, 1912).

SECONDARY SOURCES

Ackerknecht, Erwin, 'Anticontagionism between 1821 and 1867', *Bulletin of the History of Medicine* 22(5) (1948): 562–93.

Anderson, A. A., *The Book of Psalms*, vol. 2 (London: Marshall Morgan and Scott, 1981).

Bailey, Frank Edgar, *British Policy and the Turkish Reform Movement: A Study in Anglo-Turkish Relations, 1826–1853* (New York: Howard Fertig, 1970).

Baldwin, Peter, *Contagion and the State in Europe, 1830–1930* (Cambridge: Cambridge University Press, 1999).

Berkes, Niyazi, *The Development of Secularism in Turkey* (Montreal: McGill University Press, 1964).

Bowie, Walter Russell, *et al.*, *The Interpreter's Bible*. vol. 4 (Nashville, TN: Abingdon, 1939).

Bulmuş, Birsen, 'Plague in the Ottoman Empire, 1300–1838', PhD dissertation, Georgetown University, 2008.

Byrne, Joseph P., *The Black Death* (Westport, CT: Greenwood Press, 2004).

Capp, Bernard, *English Almanacs, 1500–1800: Astrology and the Popular Press* (Ithaca, NY: Cornell University Press, 1979).

Campbell, Anna, *The Black Death and Men of Learning* (New York: Columbia University Press, 1931).

Campbell, J., 'Saint Roche', *New Catholic Encyclopedia* (New York: McGraw-Hill, 1967–72), vol. 12, pp. 540–1.

Conrad Lawrence I., 'The Plague in the Early Medieval Near East', PhD dissertation, Princeton University, 1981.

Conrad, Lawrence I., 'A Ninth-century Muslim Scholar's Discussion of Contagion', in Lawrence I. Conrad and Dominik Wujastyk (eds), *Contagion: Perspectives from Pre-Modern Societies* (Aldershot: Ashgate Publishing, 2000), pp. 163–77.

Davis, Ralph, *Aleppo and Devonshire Square* (London: Macmillan, 1967).

Dols, Michael, *The Black Death in the Middle East* (Princeton, NJ: Princeton University Press, 1977).

Eisenstein, Elizabeth L., *The Printing Revolution in Early Modern Europe* (Cambridge: Cambridge University Press, 1993).

Encyclopedia of Islam, 2nd edn (Brill: Leiden, 1960–2005) (online edition). T. Fahr, 'Huruf (Ilm al-)'. Halil İnalcik, 'Bayazid II', 'Istanbul', 'The Tanzimat and its Social Effects'.

Foley, Sean, *The Arab Gulf States: Beyond Oil and Islam* (Boulder, CO: Lynne Reinner, 2010).

Foucault, Michel, *Kliniğin Doğuşu*, trans. İnci Malak Uysal (Ankara: Epos, 2002).

Gallagher, Nancy, *Medicine and Power in Tunisia, 1780–1900* (Cambridge: Cambridge University Press, 1983).

Hammer-Purgstall, Josef Freiherr von, *Geschichte des osmanischen Reiches* (Budapest, 1827).

Herlihy, David, *Black Death and the Transformation of the West* (Cambridge; MA: Harvard University Press, 1997).

İhsanoğlu, Ekmelleddin, *et al.*, *Osmanlı Tibbi Bilimler Literatürü Tarihi*, 4 vols. (İstanbul: Birmat, 2008).

İnalcık, Halil, with Donald Quataert, *An Economic and Social History of the Ottoman Empire, 1300–1914* (Cambridge: Cambridge University Press, 1994).

Ingram, John Kells, *A History of Political Economy* (New York: A. M. Kelley, 1967).

Irfan, Habib, 'Colonization of the Indian Economy, 1757–1900,' *Social Scientist* 3(8) (1975): 23–30.

Kayalı, Hasan, *Arabs and Young Turks: Ottomanism, Arabism, and Islamism in the Ottoman Empire, 1908–1918* (Berkeley, CA: University of California Press, 1997).

Keel, Othmar, *The Symbolism of the Biblical World, in Ancient Near Eastern Iconography, and The Book of Psalms* (New York: Seabury Press, 1978).

Kuhnke, LaVerne, *Lives at Risk: Public Health in Nineteenth-century Egypt* (Berkeley, CA: University of California Press, 1990).

Kürkçüoğlu, Ömer, *Osmanlı Devleti'ne Karşı Arap Bağımsızlık Hareketi (1908–1918)* (Ankara: Ankara Üniversitesi Siyasal Bilgiler Fakültesi Basın ve Yayın Yüksek Okulu Basımevi, 1982).

Latour, Bruno, *The Pasteurization of France* (Cambridge, MA: Harvard University Press, 1993).

Lewis, Bernard, *The Muslim Discovery of Europe* (New York: W. W. Norton, 1982).

Lewis, Bernard, *What Went Wrong? Western Impact and Middle Eastern Response* (Oxford: Oxford University Press, 2001).

Low, Michael C., 'Empire of the Hajj: Pilgrims, Plagues and Pan-Islam under British Surveillance, 1865–1926', MA thesis, Georgia State University, 2007.

Lowry, Heath, 'Pushing the Stone Uphill? The Impact of Bubonic Plague on Ottoman Urban Society in the Fifteenth and Sixteenth Centuries', *Journal of Ottoman Studies* 23 (2004): 93–132.

Mantran, Robert, *17. Yüzyılın İkinci Yarısında İstanbul*, vol. 1, trans. Mehmet Ali Kılıçbay and Enver Özcan (Ankara: Türk Tarih Kurumu Basımevi, 1990).

Matt, Daniel, *The Essential Kabbalah: The Heart of Jewish Mysticism* (San Francisco, CA: Harper, 1996).

Merriman, John, *A History of Modern Europe: From Renaissance to Present* (New York: Norton, 1996).

Mitchell, Timothy, *Rule of Experts: Egypt, Techno-Politics, Modernity* (Berkeley, CA: University of California Press, 2002).

Moote, A. Lloyd and Moote, Dorothy C., *The Great Plague: The Story of London's Most Deadly Year* (Baltimore, MD: Johns Hopkins University Press, 2004).

Mullett, Charles, 'The English Plague Scare of 1720–1721', *Osiris* 2 (1936): 484–516.

Mullett, Charles, 'Some Neglected Aspects of Plague Medicine in Sixteenth-century England', *Scientific Monthly* 44(4) (April, 1937): 326.

Mullett, Charles, 'Politics, Economics and Medicine: Charles Maclean and Anti-Contagionism', *Orisis* 10 (1952): 224–51.

Murphey, Rhoads, *Ottoman Warfare, 1500–1700* (New Brunswick, NJ: Rutgers University Press, 1999).

Newman, Lex, 'Epistemology of René Descartes', *Stanford Encyclopedia of Philosophy* (online edition).

Norman, York, 'Are Muslims "Jews" or "Gypsies"? A Reassessment of Bosnian Muslim Political Thought under the Habsburgs', unpublished manuscript, 2010.

Nutton, Vivian, 'Seeds of Disease: An Explanation of Contagion and Infection from the Greeks to the Renaissance', *Medical History* 27(1) (1983): 1–34.

Nutton, Vivian, 'The Reception of Fracastoro's Theory of Contagion: The Seed that Fell among Thorns?', *Osiris*, 2nd ser. 6 (1990): 196–234.

Nutton, Vivian, 'Books, Printing and Medicine in the Renaissance', *Medicina Nei Secoli Arte e Scienza* 17(2) (2005): 434–5.

Ochsenwald, William, *The Hijaz Railway* (Charlottesville, VA: University Press of Virginia, 1980).

Özbek, Nadir, 'The Politics of Welfare: Philanthropy, Voluntarism and Legitimacy in the Ottoman Empire, 1876–1914', PhD dissertation, State University of New York at Binghamton, 2001.

Panzac, Daniel, *La Peste dans l'Empire Ottoman, 1700–1850* (Leuven: E. Peeters, 1985).

Pistor-Hatam, Anja, 'Pest und Cholera: Die Wahlfahrt zu den Heilegen Stätten im Irak als gesundheitspolitisches Problem im 19. Jahrhundert', *Die Welt des Islams*, new ser. 31(2) (1991): 228–45.

Perowne, J. J. Stewart, *The Book of the Psalms: A New Translation with the Introductions and Notes Explanatory and Critical*, vol. 2 (Ann Arbor, MI: Zondervan, 1966).

Peters, John P., *The Psalms as Liturgies* (New York: Macmillan, 1922).

Porter, Roy, *The Greatest Benefit to Mankind: A Medical History of Humanity from Antiquity to the Present* (New York: Norton, 1998).

Porter, Roy, *The Creation of the Modern World: The Untold Story of the British Enlightenment* (New York: Norton, 2000).

Quataert, Donald, *The Ottoman Empire, 1700–1922* (Cambridge: Cambridge University Press, 2000).

Rahman, Fazlur, *Health and Medicine in the Islamic Tradition: Change and Identity* (Chicago, IL: ABC International Group, 1998).

Roedell, Andrew, 'The Beasts that Perish: The Problem of Evil and the Contemplation of the Animal Kingdom in English Thought, 1660–1839', PhD dissertation, Georgetown University, 2005.

Roff, William, 'Sanitation and Security: The Imperial Powers in the Nineteenth-century Hajj', *Arabian Studies* 4 (1982): pp. 143–60.

Said, Edward, *Orientalism* (New York: Pantheon Books, 1978).

Sarıyıldız, Gülden, *Hicaz Karantina Teşkilatı (1865–1914)* (Ankara: Türk Tarih Kurumu, 1996).

Scott, James C., *Seeing like a State: How Certain Schemes to Improve the Human Condition Have Failed* (New Haven, CT: Yale University Press, 1998).

Shaw, Stanford J., *Between Old and New: the Ottoman Empire under Sultan Selim III, 1789–1807* (Cambridge, MA: Harvard University Press, 1971).

Sloan, A.W., *English Medicine in the Seventeenth Century* (Bishop Auckland: Durham Academic Press, 1996).

Smith, Pamela H., *The Business of Alchemy: Science and Culture in the Holy Roman Empire* (Princeton, NJ: Princeton University Press, 1994).

Temimi, Abdeljelil, *Le Beylik de Constantine et Ḥadj Aḥmed Bey (1830–1837)* (Tunis: Revue d'histoire maghrébine, 1978).

Ulmann, Manfred, *Islamic Medicine* (Edinburgh: Edinburgh University Press, 1978).

Uludağ, Osman Şevki, 'Osmanlı Tıp Tarihinde Reaya Hastaneleri ve İmtiyazları', *Belleten* 1(1) (1937): 279–81.

Uludağ, Osman Şevki, 'Son Kapitülasyonlardan biri Karantina', *Belleten* 1(2) (1937): 445–67.

White, Sam, *The Climate of Rebellion in the Early Modern Ottoman Empire* (Cambridge: Cambridge University Press, 2011).

Wittek, Paul, *The Rise of the Ottoman Empire* (London, 1938).

Yates, Frances, *Giordano Bruno and the Hermetic Tradition* (Chicago, IL: University of Chicago Press, 1964).

Yates, Frances, *The Occult Philosophy in the Elizabethan Age* (London: Routledge Kegan Paul, 1979).

Zürcher, Jan Erik, *Turkey: A Modern History* (London: I. B. Tauris, 2003).

INDEX

Abdulhamid II, 5
Africa, 48
Ahmed Midhat , 3, 136–8, 174
Al-Ghazali , Ebu Hamid, 3, 21, 26, 28–9, 69, 72, 74–5, 84, 106
Al-Jabarti, Abd Al-Rahman, 99–100, 112
Al-Khalidi, Ruhi, 155, 175n
Al-Khatib, Lisanaddin, 9, 42–3, 63
Al-Khatimah, Ibn, 9, 42–3, 63
Al-Yahudi, İlyas bin Abram, 2, 44, 46–7, 63, 65n, 84–5, 177
alchemy, 68
Aleppo, 51, 58
Alexandria 11, 130, 134, 139, 142, 144–5
Algeria, 2, 3, 18, 47, 64, 98–100, 102, 106–9, 123–5, 127n, 133, 178
America, 48, 50
American, 12, 54, 56, 60, 97, 101, 119, 122–3, 125, 138
Amwas Incident, 7, 25
Anatolia, 44–5, 51, 136–7, 155, 174
angel, 7, 30, 32, 34, 70, 76–8, 86
anti-Catholicism, 35, 83, 116
Arabic, 10, 11, 17, 45–7, 67n, 69–71, 73, 86, 94n
Arabs, 5–6, 10, 45, 47, 67n, 71, 85, 99, 105, 134, 149, 153–5, 158, 169, 171, 174, 179
Asia, 135
Aubert-Roche, Louis, 4, 130–5, 137, 139, 149, 178
Austrian, 2, 11, 97, 101–2, 130, 132, 144
Ayat Al-Kursi (The Throne Verse), 72

Balta Liman, 4, 64, 99, 108–9, 111
Basra, 5, 153–4, 156, 158, 171
Bašeski, Ševki, 58, 63–4, 67n
Bedouins, 5, 136, 149, 154–5, 161–4, 171, 174, 179
Beirut, 57, 136
Benghazi, 135–8, 144
Berlin to Baghdad Railway, 153
Besim Ömer, 3, 147
Bible, 31, 90
Bitlisi, İdris-i, 2–3, 15, 17–19, 21, 24–9, 34, 43–8, 63, 68–70, 84–5, 177
Britain, 48, 98, 108–9, 116, 135, 154, 156, 160, 166, 179

Cabala, 68–9, 82, 84
Cairo, 11, 39, 46, 48, 50, 57, 86, 99, 133–4
Calvinist, 77
Catholicism, 116
Central Asia, 148–9
Charles II, 30–1, 88–9, 93
China, 4, 109

cholera, 4, 10, 46, 102, 104–5, 123, 128n, 130–1, 136, 140, 142–3, 146–7, 155–7, 159–60, 162, 167, 171, 173
Christ, 30–2, 34
Christian, 16, 21, 30, 33, 35–6, 44, 47, 57, 77, 81–2, 87–9, 122, 125, 148, 154
Clemow, F. G., 155–62, 164, 166, 168–74
Clot-Bey, 127n, 130–5, 137, 139, 149, 178
Companions of Prophet Muhammad, 6, 7, 19–21, 75
Conrad, Lawrence, 6–9, 11
Constantinople Superior Health Council, 4, 99, 111, 125, 130, 136–8, 141–2, 144, 148, 155, 159, 174, 179
contagion, 7–8, 21–3, 33–4, 36, 42–3, 47, 49, 54, 57–8, 67, 87, 114–17, 132, 140, 177
  anti-contagionism, 44, 59, 63, 90–1, 104, 112–13, 117–18, 123, 139–40
  contagionism , 32–3, 39, 43, 48, 52, 59, 63–4, 90, 98, 101–3, 105, 113, 118, 120, 123, 125, 128n, 131–2, 136
corpse smuggling on Ottoman–Persian border, 156
cotton, 2, 49–57, 63, 90–1, 103, 105, 108–9, 112–13, 120, 131, 139–40, 148
Crimean War, 131, 142

Damascus, 3, 6–7, 18, 24, 25, 28, 44, 46, 85, 139, 154, 175n
DeKay, James, 60–3, 101, 104, 117–23, 125
disease, 1–4, 7–10, 12, 15–18, 20–4, 27, 29, 30–6, 39–50, 52–3, 62, 68, 71–3, 76, 79–81, 87, 92–3, 97, 100–6, 112, 115–18, 120–1, 123, 127n, 130–5, 137–9, 142–6, 148, 152, 154–8, 160, 162–3, 165, 167, 169–73, 177–9
Djebel Tor, 146
Dols, Michael, 9–11, 18, 92
Dr Bartoletti, 137–8, 140–2, 155
Dutch, 54–6, 145–6, 160, 168, 178

Ebussuud Efendi, 3, 16–17, 24–9
Egypt, 1, 4, 9, 11, 14n, 17, 30, 34, 48, 64, 67n, 86, 88–9, 97–100, 104, 111–12, 127n, 130–3, 135–7, 139, 142, 145–6, 148–9, 152, 154, 159, 168, 174, 178–9
Elizabeth I, 83, 90–1
England, 12, 16, 30, 36, 39–40, 50–3, 55–6, 58, 73, 77–8, 88, 93, 108, 113, 115–16, 123
English, 2, 12, 16, 30–6, 40, 50, 52, 54–7, 63, 68–9, 75–6, 78, 83–4, 88–9, 92–3, 113, 172, 178–9
European colonisation, 2–3, 6, 18, 35, 40, 47, 99, 100, 125, 107, 115, 131, 149, 154, 168, 173–4, 179

First World War, 6, 155, 171, 174, 179
Fracastoro, Girolamo, 39, 43, 49, 63, 177
France, 35, 39, 48, 100, 109, 116, 123, 127n, 135
French, 2, 4, 6, 10–12, 18, 47, 54, 56, 64, 91, 97, 98, 99, 100, 102, 106–10, 116, 123–5, 127n, 130–4, 136–46, 149, 152, 154, 160, 162, 168, 178–9

Gaffarel, Jacques, 86–7, 89, 92
Gallagher, Nancy, 11–12, 127n
Germans, 134, 144, 153
Germany, 43, 79, 89
Greeks, 55, 64, 112, 121, 124–5, 134, 137, 148, 159, 174

Hadis, 16–17, 20–3, 25, 27, 29
Hamdan, bin Al-Merhum Osman Hoca, 2–6, 12, 15–16, 18–19, 21–3, 25–9, 33, 36, 40, 47, 68, 97, 100, 102–13, 115, 123–5, 130, 174, 177–80
Hijaz, 5–6, 12, 146–8, 153–4, 155, 160, 162–4, 167, 169, 171, 172, 174
  Hijaz Railway, 149, 154, 160–4, 167, 175n
  Hijaz Sanitary Administration, 154–5, 163–7
Holland, 48, 54–5
Hormuz, 156

India, 4, 45, 56–7, 108–9, 146, 156, 168
International Sanitary Conferences, 4, 99, 131–2, 137–42, 144, 146, 148, 152, 154–5, 160, 168–9, 173, 178
Iraq, 5–6, 12, 67n, 149, 153–6, 158–9, 169, 171–2, 174, 179

Islam, 3, 5–6, 8–12, 15–21, 23–5, 28, 30, 35–6, 42, 44, 46, 62, 65n, 67n, 69–70, 77, 86, 88, 98, 100, 102, 106–7, 111, 119, 146, 149, 153, 158, 163, 166, 168–9, 177
Istanbul, 1, 6, 11, 13, 18, 39, 46, 52, 57, 59–63, 85, 87–8, 101–2, 105, 111–12, 120, 123–4, 136–7, 139, 142, 148, 153, 171–4, 179
Italian, 39, 41, 43, 49, 57, 110, 134, 160, 177
Italy, 43, 50, 136
İzmir (Smyrna), 39, 51, 57, 91, 121, 124, 136–7, 142–3
İzzeddin, Kasım, 5–6, 154–7, 159–71, 174, 179

Jeddah, 146, 154, 162, 164–7, 169, 171–2
Jerusalem, 78, 154
Jew, 58, 121, 124, 134
Jewish, 2, 34, 44, 65n, 69, 84, 112, 122, 154
Jinn, 7, 9, 24, 70–1, 73, 75, 77

Kamaran, 146, 162, 172
Kemp, William, 77, 79–81, 88, 91, 93
Khanikin, 156–7, 159
Kuhnke, La Verne, 11

Labads or Shibna, 157
Lady Montagu, 62
Lago, Anton, 2, 11, 97, 102, 112, 124, 126n
Lausanne Peace Conference, 174, 180
League of Nations, 172–3
Lewis, Bernard, 28n, 67n
London, 2, 31, 39, 49–50, 55–7, 60, 68, 77, 78, 80, 84, 88, 90–3, 98, 109, 113–15, 118, 131, 144, 155
Louis XIV, 89
Lowry, Heath, 9–10

Maclean, Charles, 101, 105, 109, 112–13, 115–16, 118, 121–3, 125
magic, 3, 9, 12, 68, 71–4, 79, 82–94, 177–8
Mahmud II, 2, 11, 32, 35, 45–6, 97, 102, 104, 106–11, 113, 117, 119, 123–5
Mead, Richard, 49, 51–2, 54, 57–9, 63–4, 113–16
Mecca, 3–6, 15, 18, 44, 58, 86, 124, 131, 146–9, 153–4, 162, 164, 166–8, 170–2, 179
Medaini Salih, 161
medicine, 1, 10–11, 18, 20–2, 28, 30–1, 42, 45, 54, 60, 67n, 68, 92, 104–5, 110, 112, 120, 123, 132, 134, 139
Medina, 5, 20, 25, 70, 86, 124, 146, 148, 153–4, 160, 162, 164, 166, 167, 172
Mediterranean, 6, 43, 49, 52, 55–7, 69, 86, 108, 117, 127n, 132, 135, 139, 142, 146–7
Mena, 170
Miasma, 9, 33, 43, 59, 85, 90, 177
Middle East, 153, 178–9
modernisation, 11–12, 40, 98, 112–13, 125, 178
Moses, 17, 34, 82, 84, 89
Moses Wells, 146
Muhammad Ali, 4, 11, 97, 100, 104, 111, 130, 137
Muhammad, the Prophet, 3, 6–7, 16–17, 19–27, 29, 34, 70, 75, 106, 161
Muhammed Salih, 46
Mustafa Kemal Atatürk, 174
Müstakimzade, Sa'deddin Süleyman bin Muhammed Emin, 70–1

Najaf and Karbala, 153–4, 156, 159
Nile, 56, 130–3, 135

Osman, 15–18, 20–30, 32, 35–6, 44, 102, 106–7
Ottoman, 1–6, 8–12, 15–26, 28–36, 38–40, 43–64, 67n, 68–9, 71–2, 75–6, 83–5, 87–9, 91–3, 97–102, 104–13, 117–25, 130–2, 134–49, 152–65, 167–74, 177–9
Ottoman decline, 9, 11, 135
Ottoman Empire, 2–6, 9–12, 15–16, 18, 21, 29, 35, 40, 48–51, 53–4, 57, 59–60, 62–4, 69, 84, 98–9, 101, 108–9, 111–13, 119, 122–3, 125, 135–7, 139–40, 142, 144–5, 149, 153–6, 159–60, 162–3, 168, 177, 174, 177, 179

Panzac, Daniel, 10–11, 14n
Paris, 107, 131, 141, 144, 154–5, 166, 168–9, 178
pilgrimage
  Shiite pilgrimage, 5, 153
  Sunni pilgrimage, 3–4, 18, 44, 131, 146–9, 154, 162–3, 167–9
plague, 1–12, 15–36, 39–60, 63, 67n–73, 75–85, 87, 89–94n, 97–106, 109, 111–12, 114–15, 117–18, 120–5, 127n, 128n, 130–40, 143–4, 146–9, 152–7, 159–60, 169–70, 172–3, 177–9
  Alexander Yersin, 5, 8, 147, 152
  Black Death of 1347–8, 3, 9, 40, 44, 47–9, 67n, 177
  Boccaccio, 39–42, 120, 177
  bubonic, 5, 8, 147, 152
  divine origin, 7, 18–20, 23–5, 27–8, 31, 33, 35, 58, 68, 72–3, 75–8, 81–5, 89, 93
  flight, 23–4, 27
  Florence, 40–1, 43, 58
  Great Plague of London, 2, 31, 39, 50, 56, 68, 77, 80, 90, 98, 118
  magic, 3, 9, 12, 68, 71–4, 79, 82, 83–93, 177–8
  Marseilles, 32, 39, 50, 52, 77, 98, 136
  miasmastic origin, 9, 33, 43, 59, 85, 90, 177
  plague outbreaks, 6–7, 18, 137–8, 159
  tevekkül (resignation), 15, 17
  Thucydides, 47
poor, 2–3, 5, 20, 28–9, 73, 82, 112, 114–16, 119, 121, 124, 132, 149, 153, 158–9, 167, 169, 178–9
print culture, 40, 46, 68, 92
Proust, Adrien, 144–5, 147, 162, 168
Psalm 91, 76–8, 82–4

quarantine, 1–4, 6, 10–16, 18, 21, 26, 28–30, 32, 34–6, 39–40, 44, 57, 63, 97–8, 100, 102, 104–9, 111–12, 118, 125, 128n, 130, 131, 152, 174
  land quarantine, 58–9, 64, 131, 133, 154–6, 159–62, 166, 169, 172, 174
  lazarettos, 43, 49, 52, 57, 99, 101–2, 124, 136, 140, 143, 145
  maritime quarantine, 5, 6, 10, 11, 39, 41, 43, 48–52, 54–7, 97–9, 101–4, 106, 109–13, 117, 126n, 127n, 130–2, 135–46, 148–9, 152, 161, 168, 172–4
  social disciplinary tool, 3, 29, 40, 43, 63, 83, 93, 97–100, 102, 104, 106, 109, 112–18, 120–1, 123–4, 147, 153
Quran, 6, 16–17, 19, 35, 68–70, 72–3, 84–6

Red Cross, 78, 113
religion, 17, 21, 58, 88, 105–7, 119, 153
Rome, 79
Russell, Alexander, 58
Russell, Patrick, 49, 114–15
Russian, 98, 111–12, 131–4, 144, 156, 162

Saad, Lamec, 159, 175n
Saint Roche, 77–9, 84
science, 36, 45, 67n, 68, 82, 86–7, 90, 93, 105, 110, 137
Selim the Grim, 10, 67
Selim III, 15, 32, 35, 97, 102, 106–7, 110, 123
Sharif Hussein, 162, 164, 171–2, 179
Shiites, 153, 155–6, 159, 174, 179
smallpox, 22, 44, 50, 62, 165, 173
social construction, 63
social discipline, 113, 115, 123
statesmen, 6, 12, 15, 24, 46, 50, 59, 63–4, 105–6, 121
Straits, 6, 111, 130, 136, 138, 143, 174
Suez Canal, 4–5, 131, 140, 146–7, 149, 152–3, 159–60, 173–4, 179
Süleyman the Magnificent, 10, 24
syphilis, 45, 48, 50

Takvim-i Vekayi, 18
Talat Pasha, 164
talisman, 3, 68–9, 71, 73–4, 82, 84–93
Tanzimat, 28
Taşköprüzade, Kemaleddin, 3, 9, 15, 21–3, 25, 28–9, 46, 63, 68–73, 75, 84, 177

Tholozan, Joseph-Désiré, 137, 144, 156
Tunisia, 11, 98, 111, 127n
Turhan Pasha, 3, 168
Turk, 16, 45, 52, 54, 58–9, 61–2, 105, 107–8, 117–18, 120–3, 131–2, 134, 138, 145, 155, 164, 172–4, 180
Turkey, 6, 46, 51–3, 59–60, 101, 119, 122, 135, 140, 174, 180
Turkish, 11, 145–6, 88, 92, 102, 110, 119, 136

Urquhart, David, 108–9

vaccination, 152–3, 173
  anti-plague vaccination, 147
Venice, 43, 49, 52, 57, 146, 177

Westernisation, 11, 98, 104
witches, 178

Yanbu, 154, 164, 172
Yates, Francis, 68
Young Turks, 155

Zihni Pasha, 164

EU Authorised Representative:
Easy Access System Europe Mustamäe tee 50, 10621 Tallinn, Estonia
gpsr.requests@easproject.com

Printed and bound by CPI Group (UK) Ltd, Croydon, CR0 4YY
14/09/2026
02216780-0002